The Ultimate Wh[...] Mediterranean D[...]

3 Books in 1, Lower your Blood Pressure, Cholesterol Levels and Lose Weight

By

Rina S. Gritton

Acknowledgements

This book could not have been written without the guidance and generosity of many people. To all of you who encouraged and stood by me, thank you.

Copyright © 2019 Rina S. Gritton

The author retains all rights. No part of this document may be reproduced or transmitted in any form or by any means, electronic or mechanical, including photocopying, recording, or by any information storage and retrieval system without permission in writing from the author. The unauthorized reproduction or distribution of this copyrighted work is illegal.

Disclaimer

The information contained in this material is based on years of several types of research by scientists, dieticians and other professionals in the health field. Whatever you read within the pages of this book is for purely of informational purposes only and is not to be taken as a guide for diagnosis for any psychological or medical condition, nor to treat, mitigate or prevent any disease. Do not discard the professional advice from qualified health care personnel based on the information you get from this book. This book is not intended to be, and you should decide your health based on appropriate discussions with a qualified medical doctor or healthcare professional.

Contents

The Simple Mediterranean Diet Cookbook for Beginners 7

INTRODUCTION 10

CHAPTER ONE 25

CHAPTER TWO 42

CHAPTER THREE 58

CHAPTER FOUR 75

CHAPTER FIVE 90

The Essential DASH Diet Cookbook for Beginners 102

Introduction 106

Chapter One 124

Chapter Two 139

Chapter Three 152

Chapter Four 172

Chapter Five 183

Conclusion 190

The Holistic Whole Food Diet Cookbook for Everyone 192

INTRODUCTION 197

CHAPTER ONE 211

CHAPTER TWO 219

CHAPTER THREE 229

CHAPTER FOUR 239

CHAPTER FIVE 249

CHAPTER SIX 286

CHAPTER SEVEN 299

Other Books by the Author 313

The Simple Mediterranean Diet Cookbook for Beginners

Healthy, Delicious Recipes to Lose Weight, Lower Cardiac Disease for a Lifelong Healthy Life

By

Rina S. Gritton

Acknowledgements

This book could not have been written without the guidance and generosity of many people. To all of you who encouraged and stood by me, thank you.

Copyright © 2019 Rina S. Gritton

The author retains all rights. No part of this document may be reproduced or transmitted in any form or by any means, electronic or mechanical, including photocopying, recording, or by any information storage and retrieval system without permission in writing from the author. The unauthorized reproduction or distribution of this copyrighted work is illegal.

INTRODUCTION

Research and observations over the years have concluded that people around the Mediterranean are living longer and healthier lives devoid of the common ailments plaguing folks from other parts of the world. For example, heart disease is far lower on the average in this region compared to the U.S. Why are people here not suffering from heart attacks, obesity, arthritis, etc. as much as we are? The simple answer lies in their diet and mode of lifestyle. The food particular to these countries and people is termed the Mediterranean diet

The Mediterranean Diet

It is referred to as the Mediterranean Diet Plan, and it is area specific to the people and the area around the Mediterranean. This diet in itself is not what we are used to which involves restricting and limiting the intake of certain food groups. It is not a fad that is making waves in any particular area of the world. Instead, it is a lifestyle, the way of a specific group of people who have adopted the food found in their area of the world to enjoy a wholesome lifestyle. This eating habit is not all about what is consumed, but it also involves a lifestyle filled with activity rather than been sedentary which is a common cause of the ailments plaguing us. Inhabitants of this area have the lowest recorded rates of heart disease, obesity, arthritis, Alzheimer's compared to other compared parts of the world.

It is not all about a healthy intake of a variety of different food classes, but they also exercise daily. The primary food consumed includes and not limited to, protein from plant sources, vegetables, fruit, seafood and a limited amount of beef from animal sources. The oil mainly found in the diet is of the unsaturated type which is a healthier alternative when compared to saturated fats that can clog your arteries and lead to other health issues. Oils from nuts, olive oil, and fish oil are perfect for this lifestyle.

To fully maximize the potentials that this eating habit has, you need to incorporate an exercise regime into your daily schedule. This is in a structured format called the Mediterranean Diet Pyramid. With our ever busy lifestyles, there is almost no room for a concerted form of exercise to keep our bodies fit and in tip top shape. Set a target of working out for at least 3 hours every week which may range from easy to tough workouts to get your heart pumping. Such exercises include jogging, walking briskly, some aerobics, dancing, swimming, etc. It is pertinent that you engage in sporting activities that you are passionate about and not what is in fashion which may be potentially dangerous to your body. If you decide to practice a form of exercise which your body cannot handle, you will, in the end, be defeating the purpose of the diet because you may end up injured.

Healthy Weight Maintenance

Considering that the diets of the Mediterranean are high in healthy fats, if you take in too much of it, you may find your body weight ballooning if you lose count of your total calorie intake. If your aim is to shed some excess body weight, then you should aim to reduce the portions of the concerned food class.

The Peculiarity of the Mediterranean Diet

Legumes; these include seeds and nuts which are a significant source of protein from plant sources which are highly needed in our daily meals, e.g., peanuts, black beans, etc.

Whole grains; the parts of the grain which the human body makes the most use of are germ, endosperm and the bran. All of these constituents have their various purposes and due to processing to get products such as flour for baking, pasta, etc., some of the vitality is lost. This is a significant reason why brown flour or products made from whole grain are more nutritious as they still contain most of the nutrients when compared to white flour or polished rice.

Massive amounts of olive oil are consumed in this diet type in addition to oil from fish. The oils are used as an alternative to refined and artificial unhealthy fat sources.

Vegetables and fruits are consumed in large quantities as at when they are available and when in season.

Limited amounts of dairy; your favorite milk products like heavy cream, yogurt, milk, milk products should be consumed in moderation, most often not more than three times a week.

Exercise; at most 40 minutes of light to heavy activity a day, 4 to 5 times a week.

Red Wine; when consumed with meals daily, it goes a long way in maintaining good health. At least one glass a day is considered just ok.

Water; consuming at least eight glasses of a day is useful in maintaining a healthy metabolism, flushing away toxins and generally keeping the body hydrated.

Eggs, seafood, and poultry make up a significant source of animal protein in the diet while beef is quite minimal.

Rather than making use of salt which may increase the blood pressure if not taken with caution, spices and herbs have been made use of to add flavor to the dishes.

When you take a close look at most of the diet types out there, it is not made for everyone. Folks who are having some form of health challenges, young children or the aged cannot at most times partake in such diets due to the restrictive nature.

This diet type, however, can be indulged in by all and sundry as no class of essential food item is removed. If you make it a point of duty to feast on the Mediterranean diet in your home, your children will have a higher chance of experiencing a healthy life devoid of any severe medical conditions.

Health Benefits

Studies over decades have concluded that sticking with the Mediterranean diet confers immunity from a host of diseases and generally reduced death rates in the studied population. The more you adhere to this diet form, the more the occurrences of some types of conditions will reduce. Such diseases are currently major public health concerns in most western countries. They include; irritable bowel syndrome, cardiovascular diseases, various forms of cancer, arthritis, Parkinson's disease, and a few others. A recent study carried out revealed that the subjects who were prone to having cardiovascular attack who now embraced the Mediterranean diet had an almost 32% reduction rate in the chance of coming down with a heart attack when compared to those subjects who stuck with reducing the fat intake or some other forms of diets.

The vegetables and fruits have high fiber contents, antioxidants that are the body's defense mechanism against a buildup of harmful toxins. The regular intake of fresh fruits when available in season and vegetables will reduce your chances of coming down with any life-threatening ailment significantly. The daily intake of dietary fiber goes a long way in lowering your body mass index and cholesterol.

Leguminous plants are excellent sources of protein, complex carbohydrates, minerals, etc. Constant intake of legumes brings about a reduction in type 2 diabetes, excess body weight, etc.

Seafood's such as sardine and tuna are very rich in omega-3 fatty acids, mono-saturated fatty acids which aid in the anti-clotting process of the blood and it is also an essential component in anti-inflammatory compounds. There is a reduced chance of coming down with a heart attack with the optimal intake of olive oil and foods high in omega-3 fatty acids.

Starting

Just like any endeavor that you want to begin, be it a diet, a change in your lifestyle, you may find adapting to eating in the Mediterranean style a bit hard to conform to at the beginning. This is not an absolute diet like the myriad of eating fads that are out there nowadays. This diet plan is quite flexible, and you can mix it up and design it to suit your taste. Missing out on some quantity of food classed does not necessarily mean that you have failed and it will certainly not affect your health negatively. You may begin to see giant strides in your health just by starting slowly with eating a few parts of the diet.

When you start slowly with the diet plan, your body system will have time to adapt to the new food intake gradually, and you won't be overwhelmed. If you don't take fruits regularly before, you can start with a few fruits daily in combination with vegetable and legumes all in small portions. Your exercising does not have to be heavy, and the duration too should be short. It gives you time to ease into the new routine, and changes gradually can be implemented later on.

So you have finally started on the diet plan, and you have been spending so much on designer and gourmet branded food items, and your account balance is not finding it funny at all. This is a diet plan that can be kept very simple. All you need can be found on the shelves of your neighborhood supermarkets. When you go shopping, look out for whole wheat products, e.g., whole wheat bread, pasta, brown rice, etc. do not buy white flour products or polished rice, Buy a lot of vegetables and fruits, regular bottles of red wines, extra virgin olive oil, etc.

Your Budget

With the Mediterranean diet, there are always alternatives to every food item, and there is no need for you to go overboard with stocking up your kitchen with expensive food items that have cheaper and healthier alternatives. For example, instead of buying meat which can costly, you can readily get legumes, eggs, and nuts which will do your body more healthy service. Peas, black-eyed beans, peanuts are good sources of proteins of plant origin. Yogurt maybe plain regular or Greek yogurt. The difference is only slight in the thickness, protein and calcium content. They mainly contain the same types of nutrients in slightly different proportions. So based on your financial status then, go for what will not make a huge dent to your account. With fruits and vegetables, the more you invest in purchasing them, the fewer funds you will have to buy meat, which is a good thing. Based on your location, certain fruits and vegetables will be more available in some seasons than in others. With this in mind, always maximize your consumption of such fruits when in season when they are fresher and contain a higher percentage of nutrients. When in the offseason, you can make do with canned vegetables and fruits. Go with fish that is rich in omega-3 fatty acids, fresh, smoked, frozen or canned fish; it does not matter which you consume as your access to it may be limited based on your location, time of the year, social restrictions or financial status.

Other Healthy Diets

The Dietary Means to Stop Hypertension (DASH Diet) has a lot of similarities to the Mediterranean Diet. The Mediterranean diet is however distinct with much focus placed on fruits, red wine, spices and herbs, and extra virgin olive oil. This diet is not entirely based upon our diet; physical activity, rest, sleep and a host of other vital variables also places a crucial role in the overall health of your body and mind.

Avoid

With your mind made up to start eating healthy, you will have to do away with some unhealthy foods and ingredients that will surely negate any success you could have made. Foods to be avoided;

Refined produce; any product made with refined wheat.

Refined oil; cottonseed, soybean oil, etc

Extremely processed foods;

Sugars; candies, soda drinks, white table sugar, etc.

Trans fats; any fat that has been processed and added to food products coming out of a factory.

In essence, whenever you go shopping, always read the labels of any food that you are going to buy to ensure it as natural as possible and contains little or no amount of artificial preservatives and flavoring agents.

Fluids

As with any healthy diet regime, water should be the most essential fluid that you consume. It forms the basis of your beverage drink every day. A glass of red wine every day with your meal has excellent health benefits. It is not a must that you take wine most especially if you have a challenge with alcohol or any other condition that can be exacerbated by the intake of any form of alcohol. You can take in your teas or coffees but ensure the sweetening agent is healthy, e.g., honey. Also, try to stay away from drinks and juices that are high in sugar content.

In the End

There is no apparent definition of what a Mediterranean diet is, but is indeed a way of life that involves eating healthy foods mainly of plant origins and moderate to low amounts of animal contents which are mostly seafood. All in all, this diet is a perfectly healthy choice that any family can practice and love all the way.

CHAPTER ONE
Delish

Veggie Egg Avocado

Ingredients

One large tomato, sliced

One small eggplant, thinly sliced

Three eggs, hard-boiled, sliced

Two large white onions, chopped

Two avocados, finely chopped

One small carrot, grated

½ teaspoon, fresh lemon juice

½ teaspoon cayenne

½ teaspoon dried basil

One clove garlic, minced

Two tablespoons extra virgin olive oil

A pinch of sea salt

Directions

- In a large bowl, thoroughly mix the lemon juice and avocado.

- Add all the other ingredients to a large bowl except for the tomato. Combine well.
- Serve on whole wheat bread with the tomatoes.

Greek Briam

Ingredients

2 cups extra virgin olive oil

Two large green onions, thinly sliced

Two large carrots, thinly sliced

Two medium sized aubergine

½ cup yellow corn, boiled

Four cloves garlic, crushed

1 kg large Irish potatoes, cubed

500g tomato paste

Ten large red tomatoes, sliced

½ teaspoon paprika

½ teaspoon chili

½ teaspoon black pepper

½ teaspoon oregano

Directions

- Preheat the oven to 235°C
- Slice the aubergine into thick slices
- Cook the aubergine over medium heat in olive oil for 6 – 8 minutes. Add oil as you deem fit. Move to a large bowl.
- To a new pan, sauté sliced onions and garlic in olive oil until brown. Pour contents into the bowl with the aubergine.
- Combine the potatoes, paste, yellow corn, tomatoes and 210 ml of water into a bowl.
- Add the spices and mix well using your hands. Pour into an ovenproof dish.
- Apply olive oil over the mixture.
- Bake for 25 minutes at 235°C then reduce the temperature to 195°C and bake for another 15 minutes.
- Serve after cooling a bit.

Portobellos

Eight large Portobello mushrooms, gills removed and cleaned

Four large tomatoes, sliced

2 cups, mozzarella, shredded

Olive oil

½ teaspoon black pepper

One clove garlic, crushed

Directions

- Preheat the oven to 250°C.
- Apply a baking sheet into the baking pan.
- Sprinkle the mushroom with olive oil and the spices.
- Add in the sliced tomatoes and dowse with some olive oil too.
- Sprinkle the cheese over the mixture.
- Let the mixture sit and marinate for a few minutes.
- Bake until the mushroom is cooked.
- Serve warm

Lemony Medi Soup with Quinoa

Ingredients

2 cups boiled quinoa

One large onion, thinly sliced

Four garlic cloves, crushed

2 cups extra virgin olive oil

½ cup fresh lemon juice

½ teaspoon chili

½ teaspoon thyme

½ teaspoon oregano

½ teaspoon paprika

½ teaspoon curry

5 cups vegetable broth

1 ½ cup water

3 cups heavy cream

Sea salt

Directions

- Preheat the oven to 250°C.
- Pour in the quinoa onto a baking sheet placed in a pan. Sprinkle the spices on salt over it. Drizzle with olive oil.
- Mix thoroughly.

- Bake for 35 minutes.
- Sautee onions and garlic with olive oil over medium heat in a large pot. Stir for about 2 minutes.
- Add some of the quinoa and stir well.
- Add the broth and water.
- Allow to boil, and then let it simmer for about 10 minutes.
- Take off heat and blend mixture using a hand-held blender.
- Put back the mixture on heat and pour in the heavy cream and lemon juice and add the remaining quinoa.
- Stir the quinoa well and cook for about 2 minutes.
- Add some salt as you desire.
- Serve hot with garlic bread.

Mediterranean Zucchini Roll-Ups

Ingredients

One large zucchini

½ teaspoon cayenne pepper

¼ teaspoon garlic powder

Five tablespoon hummus

1 cup dried tomatoes, chopped

1 cup feta cheese, crumbled

Sea salt

Directions

- Peel off long thin slices of the zucchini using a vegetable peeler.
- Sprinkle the slices with the pepper.
- Spread hummus on each slice.
- Add the chopped smoked tomatoes and cheese on each slice.
- Roll the zucchini from one end to the other encompassing the filling.
- Make the roll firm and secure using a toothpick.
- Serve and enjoy.

Chicken with Tzatziki Sauce

Tzatziki Sauce

One large cucumber, cleaned and cubed

Five cloves garlic, minced

One small red onion, thinly sliced

½ teaspoon black pepper

Two tablespoons lemon juice, fresh

½ cup fresh dill

1 cup olive oil

Sea salt

Chicken

Six chicken breasts pounded to a 1-inch thickness

One green bell pepper, thinly sliced

1 ½ tablespoon Italian seasoning

One large white onion, thinly sliced

Six pitas

1 cup feta cheese

Directions

- Pour all the ingredients for the sauce into a high powered food blender. Blend until smooth and cover until ready for use.

- Season the chicken using the Italian seasoning and spices.
- Cook over heat in olive oil until each side is brown.
- Remove from heat and allow cooling.
- Cut into strips.
- Spread out the pitas, lay out the chicken strips on the bread, apply the sauce and feta cheese and roll it up or fold.

Sardinian Grilled Chicken

Ingredients

2 pounds boneless, skinless chicken breasts, cubed

½ cup extra virgin olive oil

½ teaspoon paprika

One teaspoon oregano

½ teaspoon jalapeno

Three cloves garlic, minced

Two tablespoon lemon juice, fresh

One bowl of fresh olives

One red bell pepper, thinly sliced

One large red onion, thinly sliced

½ teaspoon dried basil

Sea salt

Directions

- Combine all the individual spices in a large bowl and mix thoroughly.
- Skewer the chicken and alternate with the olives.
- Place the skewed chickens into a baking pan.
- Drizzle the marinade sauce over the chicken and let it marinade for about 16 – 24 hours.
- Take the skewers out of the sauce and season with some salt.
- Grill the chicken until cook to your desired taste.
- Drizzle the chicken with lemon juice and olive oil if needed.
- Serve warm and enjoy.

Dill Yogurt and Smoked Chicken

Smoked Chicken

Ten boneless, skinless chicken thighs

Eight tablespoons extra virgin olive oil

½ teaspoon oregano

½ teaspoon paprika

Two cloves garlic, crushed

One small onion, thinly sliced

½ teaspoon black pepper

½ teaspoon Italian seasoning

½ cup lemon juice, freshly squeezed

Yogurt Sauce

2 cups fresh dill, chopped

Two tablespoons olive oil

2 cups Greek yogurt

Two cloves garlic, crushed

½ cup lemon juice

1/2teaspoon basil

Directions

- To prepare the yogurt sauce, combine all the sauce ingredients and pour into a high powered food processor. Blitz at high speed until the desired consistency has been achieved. Pour into a small bowl and refrigerate.
- To another small bowl, add the spices, some garlic and olive oil. Dip the chicken into this mixture and cover entirely with the mixture.
- To a large bowl, spread some sliced onions. Place the spiced chicken onto the onions, drizzle some olive oil and lemon juice over it.
- Seal the bowl and make airtight. Let it sit and marinate for a minimum of 12 hours in the fridge.
- Turn on the grill and smoke your chicken on each side until well done.
- Serve the smoked chicken with the yogurt dip and some salad.

Athenian Spinach, black-eyed peas and potatoes Soup

Ingredients

Four medium sized potatoes, cleaned and cubed

Two large carrots, cubed

Three cloves garlic, minced

4 cups spinach, chopped

One large onion, thinly sliced

One teaspoon black pepper

Four tablespoons extra virgin olive oil

1 cup kale, chopped

6 cups vegetable broth

Two large tomatoes, sliced

One large green bell pepper, sliced

2 cups beans, cooked

1 cup feta cheese, crumbled

½ teaspoon oregano

½ tablespoon lemon juiced

½ teaspoon basil

Sea salt

Directions

- In a large pan and over medium heat, sauté the carrots, onions, and garlic for about 4 minutes in olive oil.
- Add in the vegetables, potatoes, broth, and spices. Stir well.
- Allow cooking over medium heat for about 25 minutes.
- Add the spinach and kale and cook for another 10 minutes.
- Stir well and add the lemon juice.
- Let it simmer for about 1 minute.
- Serve warm with feta cheese.

Spicy Mushroom Kabobs

Ingredients

2 pounds mushrooms

½ cup apple cider vinegar

Two cloves garlic, minced

One small onion, thinly sliced

½ teaspoon allspice

½ teaspoon black pepper

Sea salt

Directions

- Preheat oven to 250°C.
- Coat baking pan with nonstick spray.
- Thoroughly mix the olive oil, spices in a bowl.
- Add the mushrooms and mix well. Let it marinate for about 30 minutes.
- Skewer the mushrooms and place onto the baking pan.
- Roast for about 20 minutes
- Serve hot with a side dish.

Florentine Salad with Avocado

Ingredients

1 pound big tomatoes, sliced

Three medium-sized cucumbers, sliced

1 cup extra virgin olive oil

One large onion, sliced

Three cloves garlic, crushed

2 cups feta cheese, crumbled

Three avocados, cut into chunks

1 cup apple cider vinegar

½ teaspoon black pepper

½ teaspoon paprika

½ teaspoon oregano

1 cup olives, halved

Three teaspoons sugar

Sea salt

Directions

- Pour in the vinegar, olive oil, garlic, sugar and other spices to a jar. Seal and shake very well.
- Into a mixing bowl, add the tomatoes, onion, olives, cucumber. Toss well. Put the avocado into another bowl and keep.
- Add two tablespoons of the dressing sauce to the avocado and mix gently.
- Add the remaining dressing to the salad

mixture and combine thoroughly. Add in the avocado and feta cheese.
- Serve and enjoy.

CHAPTER TWO

Dinners

Roasted Chicken with Kale and Asparagus

Three tablespoons extra virgin olive oil

Eight pieces chicken thighs

Two tablespoons butter

One large white onion, thinly sliced

2 cups asparagus, chopped

½ teaspoon cumin

½ teaspoon chili

One large green bell pepper, sliced

2 cups vegetable broth

4 cups kale, chopped

One clove garlic, minced

Two large carrots, thinly sliced

½ teaspoon ginger powder

Sea salt

Directions

- Preheat oven to 275°C
- Add the olive oil and butter to an oven-safe saucepan.
- Season the chicken with some of the spices.
- Add the skin to the butter and olive oil. Cook each side for about 8 minutes each.
- Remove the chicken from the oil and set aside.
- Add the asparagus, carrots, onions, garlic and other spices to the oil.
- Sauté for 7 minutes. Stir continuously.
- Add the kale and sauté for another 2 minutes.
- Take off heat and add the chicken and broth.
- Place the pan into the oven and oven bake for 25 minutes.
- Remove from the oven and allow o cool for about 10 minutes.
- Serve immediately.

Creamy Brussels Sprout and Salmon

Ingredients

1 ½ fresh Brussels sprouts

12 salmon filet

Three cloves garlic, minced

One large carrot, sliced

2 cups heavy cream

Two tablespoons Dijon mustard

½ teaspoon oregano

½ teaspoon thyme

One teaspoon allspice

One small onion, thinly sliced

1 cup extra virgin olive oil

Sea salt

Directions

- Preheat oven to 275°C
- Cook sprouts and carrots for about 5 minutes in 1 cup of water. Strain.
- Add the olive oil to a large saucepan and cook the salmon over medium heat for

- about 5 minutes on each side.
- Introduce the sprouts and carrots and cook for 2 minutes. Stir continuously.
- Add some of the cheese, cream, mustard, and spices to a bowl and combine well.
- Remove the cooking pan off the heat and pour in the cream sauce over the asparagus. Top with the remaining cheese.
- Arrange into the oven and bake for about 20 minutes.
- Take out from the oven and let it cool for some minutes.
- Serve warm.

Quinoa Stuffed Bell Peppers

Ingredients

2 cups quinoa

Eight green peppers

Two large tomatoes, sliced

One large red onion, thinly sliced

3 cups vegetable broth

One tablespoon butter

½ teaspoon chili

½ teaspoon black pepper

2 cups yellow sweet corn

One large carrot, grated

3 cups parmesan and cheddar cheese

1 cup yogurt

1 cup brown beans

One clove garlic, minced

½ teaspoon cilantro

Sea salt

Directions

- Preheat the oven to 275°C.
- Slice the bell peppers in half and deseed.
- Use the butter to grease the baking pan.
- Pour in the broth and quinoa into a saucepan and bring to boil; reduce the heat and let it simmer and cook for about

20 minutes.
- Take the pan off the heat.
- Pour in some olive oil into a pan and heat over medium heat.
- Sauté the onions and garlic for 2 minutes over medium heat.
- Add in the beans and corns and stir continuously for another 3 minutes.
- Add the quinoa and tomatoes with spices.
- Add some of the cheese and stir well. Cook for 5 minutes.
- Fill the bell peppers with the quinoa mixture.
- Bake for 35 minutes.
- Remove the baking pan out of the oven and top each bell pepper with some of the cheese.
- Put back into your oven and bake for 3 minutes.
- Take pan out of the oven and allow cooling.
- Serve a dash of yogurt.

Smoked Turkey Pasta Alfredo

Ingredients

2 pounds boneless, skinless smoked turkey breasts

500g pasta

Four tablespoons flour

1 cup low-fat yogurt

1 ½ cup vegetable broth

½ cup chicken broth

One clove garlic, minced

Four tablespoons olive oil

One small onion, thinly sliced

½ teaspoon cilantro

½ teaspoon black pepper

Sea salt

Directions

- Sauté garlic and onions in olive oil over medium heat.
- Add the flour and stir well.

- Add the chicken and vegetable broths.
- Cook until desired consistency is achieved.
- Add the cheese and spices. Stir thoroughly.
- Cook the pasta by boiling with some salt or by following the directions on the pack.
- Pour the prepared sauce over the pasta and using a wooden spoon, combine well.
- Serve warm with the smoked turkey.

Sicilian Pasta

Ingredients

4 cups vegetable broth

1 cup chicken broth

1 cup kale, chopped

Two large tomatoes, sliced

1 ½ pound pasta

Four cloves garlic, crushed

One teaspoon allspice

½ teaspoon jalapeno

Four tablespoons extra virgin olive oil

1 cup mixed cheese

½ teaspoon paprika

Sea salt

Directions

- To a pot, add the pasta, broth, spices, tomatoes, and salt.
- Cook until the mixture begins to boil.
- Simmer on low heat for 12 - 15 minutes. Stir continuously.
- Take off heat and allow to cool.
- Add the cheese and combine well.
- Serve warm and enjoy.

Galleon Chicken Wings and Veggies

Ingredients

Six chicken wings

Six tablespoons extra virgin olive oil

Three cloves garlic, minced

Six large aluminum foils

One green bell pepper, sliced

One white onion, sliced

½ cup parsley leaves, chopped

½ teaspoon basil

½ teaspoon coriander

One teaspoon allspice

½ cup chicken dressing

Two medium-sized carrots, chopped

Sea salt

Directions

- Preheat oven to 250°C.
- Arrange the chicken wings individually on the foils.
- Dowse with olive oil.
- Sprinkle the spices all over the chicken.
- Put the onions, carrots, pepper, and garlic all around and on top of the wings.
- Apply the dressing over the chicken.
- Cover the chicken tightly with the foil.
- Place the foils in a baking pan.

- Bake for 40 – 45 minutes.
- Take the chicken from the oven and allow to cool for 5 minutes.
- Serve immediately.

Zucchini and Cheddar One-Pot Pasta

Ingredients

500g pasta

Four tablespoons extra virgin olive oil

5 cups water

6 cups zucchini, chopped

Four cloves garlic

One medium sized onion, chopped

One large red bell pepper, sliced

½ teaspoon cumin

½ teaspoon basil

½ teaspoon chili

½ teaspoon allspice

1 cup cheddar cheese

Sea salt

Directions

- Heat some oil over low to medium heat in a pot.
- Add the zucchini and a pinch of salt. Sauté for about 3 minutes.
- Take it off heat and add the remaining ingredients.
- Cook on high heat until it begins to boil.
- Turn the heat and let it simmer for another 10 minutes.
- Take it off the heat and all to cool.
- Add some olive oil and cheese.
- Stir well and serve.

Slow Cooker Eggplant and Carrot Soup

Ingredients

Two large eggplants, thinly sliced

Six large carrots, cubed

2 cups kale, chopped

1 cup yellow corn, boiled

8 cups chicken broth

One large onion, chopped

One clove garlic, minced

1 cup spinach, chopped

One teaspoon allspice

½ teaspoon black pepper

Sea salt

Directions

- Arrange all the ingredients into the slow cooker.
- Pour in the broth.
- Seal the pot and cook on high heat setting for 4 – 5 hours.
- Use a hand-held blender to puree the soup one cup at a time.
- Serve warm with some brown rice or garlic bread.

Slow Cooker Duck Chili

Ingredients

2 cups black-eyed peas, drained and rinsed

Four large tomatoes, sliced

2 cups sweet corn

½ teaspoon parsley

One clove garlic, minced

One large red onion, chopped

½ teaspoon chili

One teaspoon allspice

¼ teaspoon oregano

2 pounds boneless duck breast

One teaspoon ginger, grated

½ cup white wine

1 cup mixed cheese

2 cups vegetable broth

½ cup heavy cream

½ teaspoon thyme

Sea salt

Directions

- Put the corn, tomatoes, beans, onions into

the slow cooker.
- Add in the spices.
- Pour in the broth and wine.
- Add the duck.
- Cover the pot and cook on high heat setting for 6 – 8 hours.
- Take out the duck and allow cooling.
- Shred the duck with a fork and return to the pot.
- Cook for another 20 minutes.
- Serve warm with heavy cream and cheese toppings.

Spicy Shrimp and Kale with Macaroni

500g Macaroni

One large white onion, chopped

Two tablespoons butter

2 pounds raw shrimp, cleaned

Three tablespoons extra virgin olive oil

Two large tomatoes, sliced

One teaspoon ginger, grated

2 cups kale, chopped

½ teaspoon chili

½ teaspoon garlic powder

One teaspoon allspice

Sea salt

Directions

- Prepare the macaroni following the instructions on the pack.
- Sauté the shrimp, onions, tomatoes, and spices in olive oil for about 5 minutes.
- Add in the kale, stir continuously and cook for another 2 minutes.
- Add the macaroni and combine well.
- Serve immediately.

CHAPTER THREE
Elevate

Tuscan Guacamole

Three large avocados pitted and halved

Four tablespoons diced tomato

¼ teaspoon paprika

½ teaspoon oregano

½ teaspoon black pepper

One medium sized onion, chopped

2 ½ tablespoon lemon juice

Two tablespoon sun-dried tomatoes, chopped

One tablespoon, extra virgin olive oil

Sea salt

Directions

- Pour the lemon juice and avocado into a mixing bowl and combine thoroughly until a fine paste is obtained.
- Add the remaining spices and mix well.
- Serve and enjoy with your choice of a

dish!

Egg Muffins with Bacon

Ingredients

12 bacon slices

½ cup eggplant, thinly sliced

½ cup mixed cheese

One medium sized onion, chopped

One clove garlic, minced

One large tomato, chopped

½ teaspoon oregano

½ teaspoon thyme

¼ teaspoon curry

¼ teaspoon black pepper

Six large organic eggs

Sea salt

Directions

- Apply cooking spray to the muffin tin. Preheat oven to 315°C.

- Lay each tin with bacon strips to entirely cover the insides.
- Apply some of the spices to each of the tin.
- Whisk the egg in a bowl with some of the spices.
- Pour the eggs into the muffin tins.
- Bake for 12 – 15 minutes.
- Remove from oven and allow cooling for 2 minutes.
- Serve immediately.

Herculean Omelette

Ingredients

14 large organic eggs

3 cups whole milk

One clove garlic, minced

Three tablespoons olive oil

½ teaspoon chili

¼ teaspoon ginger powder

1 cup spinach, chopped

1 cup asparagus, chopped

One large green bell pepper, sliced

1 cup feta cheese, crumbled

One teaspoon, fresh lemon

Sea salt

Directions

- Preheat oven to 280°C.
- Sauté the pepper, onions, asparagus, spinach, garlic in olive oil over medium heat for about 2 minutes.
- Spread the sautéed vegetables into the baking pan.
- In another bigger bowl, beat the eggs with the lemon and spices.
- Pour the egg into the baking pan with the vegetables.
- Add the crumbled cheese over the egg.
- Bake for 30 – 40 minutes.
- Serve warm.

Cheddar Frozen Yoghurt

Ingredients

2 cups full cream Greek yogurt

1 cup cheddar cheese

¼ teaspoon nutmeg

¼ teaspoon cinnamon

One tablespoon honey

Directions

- Pour all the ingredients into a blender.
- Blitz at high speed for about 2 minutes.
- Pour into a wide flat bowl.
- Put into a freezer for about 8 hours until frozen.
- Take out the frozen yogurt and break it. Return it into the blender with some milk.
- Blend until smooth.
- Serve with honey toppings.

Spartan Goddess Bowl

Ingredients

1 cup kale, chopped

1 cup eggplant, chopped

One large tomato, sliced

Two carrots, thinly sliced

1 cup green peas, cleaned

½ teaspoon oregano

¼ teaspoon cilantro

½ teaspoon paprika

One clove garlic, minced

One teaspoon ginger, grated

One tablespoon extra virgin olive oil

One tablespoon honey

One tablespoon lemon juice

Sea salt

Directions

- Preheat oven to 295°C.
- Add peas, spices, honey, and salt to a large bowl. Toss well.
- Grease baking pan and add the peas to the pan. Bake for 25 to 35 mins. Remove

from the oven and keep.
- To another bowl. Add the kale, eggplant, carrot and lemon juice and combine well.
- Top the peas with the kale salad.
- Serve immediately with your choice of dressing.

Garlic Bread Quinoa with Banana

Ingredients

4 cups very ripe bananas, mashed

1 ½ cup quinoa

½ cup crushed walnuts

Two cloves garlic, minced

½ teaspoon nutmeg

½ teaspoon cinnamon

3 cups full cream milk

One tablespoon chocolate powder

½ teaspoon ginger, grated

One teaspoon allspice

½ cup brown sugar

¼ cup honey

Sea salt

Directions

- Add the mashed banana, quinoa, chocolate powder, ginger, garlic, and spices. Combine thoroughly until all ingredients are evenly distributed.
- Add in the full cream milk and stir it properly.
- Seal the bowl airtight and refrigerate for at least 12 hours.
- Preheat oven to 285°C.
- Mix the banana mixture well again and pour in the dough into a well greased baking pan.
- Seal the baking pan with foil and bake for 65 – 90 minutes.
- Sprinkle the crushed walnuts over the baking banana mixture. Bake for 5 minutes.
- Lift the baking pan out of the oven and let

it cool for a few minutes.
- Serve warm.

Tuscan Salad

Ingredients

One large zucchini thinly sliced lengthwise

1 cup full cream Greek yogurt

One teaspoon ginger, grated

Two cloves garlic, crushed

One teaspoon cilantro

One medium sized onion, chopped

½ teaspoon black pepper

½ teaspoon nutmeg

½ cup feta cheese, crumbled

One medium-sized bell pepper, thinly sliced

One teaspoon parsley

Sea salt

Directions
- Lay the thin slices of the zucchini on a

flat, clean surface.
- To a bowl, add the other ingredients and combine well.
- Apply some of the sauce on each slice of zucchini. Sprinkle some cheese and roll the zucchini lightly.

Corsican Tuna Salad

Ingredients

500g tuna, drained

½ tablespoon, cilantro

½ tablespoon parsley

1 cup lettuce, chopped

½ cup carrot, thinly sliced

One small onion, chopped

Three tablespoons extra virgin olive oil

½ tablespoon lemon juice

Ten olives, pitted and sliced

½ teaspoon black pepper

One tablespoon capers

Directions

- Toss and combine all the ingredients in a large mixing bowl.
- Break the tuna using a fork.
- Serve immediately and enjoy.

Melon Pizzarita

Ingredients

One large Watermelon

Eight olives, pitted and sliced

One tablespoon balsamic glaze

½ teaspoon cilantro

½ teaspoon mint leaves

1 cup feta cheese, crumbled

Directions

- Cut the watermelon in half.
- Cut a 1 ½ inch slice from the half and cut each slice into wedges.
- Arrange the wedges on a large flat dish.
- Top the wedges with the glaze, olives,

cilantro, mint leaves, and cheese.
- Serve and enjoy.

Greek Scrambled Eggs

Ingredients

Six large organic eggs

One large white onion, chopped

One clove garlic, minced

Two tablespoons extra virgin olive oil

Four large tomatoes, slices

One teaspoon allspice

1/2 cup spinach, chopped

½ teaspoon chili

½ teaspoon oregano

Sea salt

Directions

- Sauté the onions and garlic in olive oil over medium heat in a large saucepan for 2 minutes.
- Add the other spices and ingredients.

- Stir well and cook for 1 minute.
- Crack the organic eggs into the saucepan and stir continuously until adequately cooked.
- Serve warm and enjoy.

Stuffed Potatoes with Brown Beans and Tahini Sauce

Ingredients

12 large Irish potatoes, cleaned and washed

Brown Beans

2 cups brown beans, cooked

One clove garlic, minced

One small onion, chopped

½ teaspoon paprika

½ tablespoon oregano

½ tablespoon lemon juice

Four tablespoons extra virgin olive oil

One tablespoon cilantro

Sea salt

Tahini Sauce

½ cup tahini sauce

½ cup water

One tablespoon fresh cilantro

½ tablespoon fresh parsley

½ tablespoon lemon juice, fresh

Directions

- Preheat oven to 325°C
- Using a fork, make holes in the potatoes and place on a baking sheet.
- Bake for 50 to 60 minutes.
- Add the ingredients for the brown beans in a large bowl. Toss well, seal and keep to one side.
- Add all the ingredients needed for the sauce into a high powered food processor. Blitz at high speed for 2 minutes or until desired consistency is achieved. Gently drain the contents of the blender into a bowl.

- Remove the potatoes from the oven and allow cooling. Cut in half and fill with the beans mixture: top with tahini sauce and some cheese.
- Best served immediately.

Quinoa, Brussels Sprouts with Hummus

Ingredients

2 cups quinoa, divided

Four tablespoons extra virgin olive oil

2 cups Brussels sprouts

One large onion, chopped

Two cloves garlic

½ teaspoon black pepper

One teaspoon allspice

Hummus

Sea salt

Directions

- Preheat oven to 325°C.
- Rinse and clean the quinoa. Dry using a

paper towel.
- Pour 1 cup into the bowl and add a tablespoon full of olive oil. Toss well.
- Pour the mixture into a large baking pan and spread evenly.
- Sprinkle some pepper and salt over it.
- Bake for 25 to 30 minutes and stir occasionally.
- Remove the baked quinoa from the oven and allow to cool. Pour into a blender and crush it. Do not blend it into flour.
- Sauté the onions and garlic in olive oil over medium heat for 2 minutes. Add the sprouts and stir for another 2 minutes.
- Pour the sprout mixture into the food processor and add the other cup of quinoa. Blend at high speed until creamy smooth.
- Pour the sprout mixture into a bowl and add the quinoa crumbs. Stir well until it is well combined.
- Form sizeable patties from the "dough."

- Grease the saucepan with some olive oil and cook the patties for about 2 minutes on each side.
- Serve warm with some hummus and enjoy!

CHAPTER FOUR
Lunch

Tangiers Lettuce Wraps

Ingredients

Ten large lettuces

One large carrot, grated

One sizeable green bell paper, thinly sliced

½ cup walnuts, crushed

Two tablespoons honey

½ cup extra virgin olive oil

One tablespoon cilantro

½ teaspoon oregano

One tablespoon parsley

Two tablespoons tahini

One tablespoon lemon juice

2 cups green peas

½ cup eggplant, thinly sliced

½ teaspoon allspice

Sea salt

Directions

- Add the peas, honey, lemon juice, tahini, vegetables and other spices to a bowl. Toss to combine well.
- Ladle the mixture onto the lettuce leaves. Sprinkle some walnuts, cilantro, and parsley on it. Secure the sheets around the dough.
- Serve and enjoy.

Chicken Flax Bowl

Ingredients

2 pounds chicken thighs

Eight tablespoons extra virgin olive oil

Four tomatoes, roasted and shredded

One large yellow bell pepper, sliced

½ teaspoon chili

One large onion, chopped

Two cloves garlic, crushed

Eight olives, pitted and chopped

½ cup feta cheese

½ teaspoon oregano

½ teaspoon paprika

1 cup carrot, thinly sliced

½ cup kale

½ teaspoon basil

1 cup flax seeds, cooked

Sea salt

Directions

- Preheat oven to 245°C.
- Spice the chicken thighs. Set it on greased baking foil.
- Place the chicken thighs in the oven and bake for 50 to 60 minutes.
- Remove chicken from the oven and all to cool.
- Shred the meat using a fork.
- Place the flax seeds, olive oil, and onions in a bowl. Combine well.

- Add the spices, olive oil, vegetables and peppers to a blender. Blitz at high speed until creamy.
- Serve the flax in bowls with the chicken and the spicy sauce.

Sanremo Lunch Pack

Ingredients

Four garlic bread sticks halved

Four slices eggplant

Two olives pitted and halved

Two slices capocollo

1 cup grapes

Cheese

Directions

- Cut each slice of capocollo lengthwise.
- Wrap each slice with some cheddar cheese.
- Place the wrapped cheese, eggplant, olives, breadsticks and grapes in Ziploc bags or airtight containers.

- Refrigerate and consume during your lunch.

Arugula Salad

Ingredients

3 cups arugula

One medium sized onion, chopped

Two tablespoons extra virgin olive oil

¼ teaspoon black pepper

Two tablespoons feta cheese

One large tomato, sliced

One tablespoon apple cider vinegar

Two tablespoons hummus

Directions

- Add all the different parts to a large bowl.
- Toss to combine well.
- Serve or refrigerate.
- Enjoy with some smoked chicken or bread.

Maroc Wrap

Ingredients

½ cup couscous

½ cup parsley, chopped

Two cloves garlic, minced

¾ cup water

1 ½ pound boneless lamb chops, cubed

Four tablespoons lemon juice, fresh

1 ½ cup cucumber, chopped

Four tablespoons extra virgin olive oil

One large tomato, chopped

One small onion, chopped

One teaspoon allspice

½ teaspoon basil

Sea salt

Five pita bread

Directions

- Pour the water into a saucepan and boil. Add the couscous and stir for about a minute. Take off the heat and allow

cooling for 3 minutes. Stir and set it aside.
- To a bowl, add the pepper, olive oil, lemon juice, basil, parsley, onions and garlic, and other spices. Combine well.
- Add about two tablespoons of the basil mixture to the lamb chops in a bowl. Combine thoroughly using your hands.
- Add some tablespoons of olive oil to a saucepan and cook the lamb chops over medium heat for about 10 - 15 minutes while stirring continuously.
- Add the remaining basil mixture to the couscous with the tomato and cucumber.
- Spread the couscous onto each of the pita bread followed by the lamb chops. Roll up the bread with some foil to securely hold the fillings in place.
- Enjoy!

Tarragona Bento Lunch

Ingredients

½ cup lentil, rinsed and drained

500g smoked chicken breast

½ cup zucchini

One tablespoon basil

One teaspoon white-wine vinegar

One tablespoon extra virgin olive oil

Two tablespoons feta cheese, crumbled

½ cup tomato, chopped

Eight olives pitted and halved

½ cup grapes

Two tablespoons tahini

½ teaspoon allspice

Sea salt

Directions

- Into a bowl, add the lentils, basil, vinegar, cheese, olives, zucchini, and other ingredients. Toss and combine well.
- Add the chopped chicken breast to a container and seal.
- To another small container, add the

tahini, olives, and grapes.
- Enjoy!

Cartagena Tuna Salad

Ingredients

1kg tuna, cleaned and drained

Four tablespoons extra virgin olive oil

2 cups asparagus, chopped

Four large tomatoes, sliced

One clove garlic, minced

1 cup lentils, drained and rinsed

½ teaspoon black pepper

One tablespoon lemon juice

½ teaspoon allspice

Sea salt

Directions

- Combine the lentils, tuna, asparagus, lemon, and spices. Put in a container and refrigerate.
- Serve slightly chill and enjoy.

Florentine Veggies

Ingredients

2 cups cauliflower

2 ½ tablespoons vinegar

2 cups leeks, chopped

One large tomato, sliced

Two tablespoons extra virgin olive oil

½ teaspoon paprika

½ teaspoon basil

Eight slices whole wheat bread

½ cup cheddar cheese

Directions

- Add the chopped onions to some cold water for a few minutes and then dry using a paper towel.
- Add the other ingredients to a bowl and combine.
- Spread the cheese over the slices of bread followed by the cauliflower mixture.

- Apply the onions, tomatoes, and leek.
- Cover up the bread with another slice.
- Enjoy immediately.

Tuna Pita Sandwich

Ingredients

5 ounces tuna, flaked

Six slices whole wheat bread

One teaspoon lemon juice, fresh

Three tablespoons Greek yogurt

One tablespoon dill, chopped

½ teaspoon oregano

½ teaspoon basil

Directions

- Combine and toss all the different ingredients in a bowl except for the bread.
- Apply the mixture generously to a side of sliced bread and then cover it with the other half.
- Pack in your lunch box and enjoy!

Veal, Mozzarella and Baguette

Ingredients

Eight slices, whole wheat baguette

Six mozzarella balls

One large tomato, sliced

½ cup olives pitted and halved

½ cup almonds, roasted and crushed

Six slices veal thinly cut

½ teaspoon allspice

Directions

- Combine all the ingredients but the bread in a bowl.
- Remove the soft inner part of the baguette.
- Spread the mixture evenly over the baguette.
- Pack in foils or sealable containers.
- Enjoy!

Sunshine Pasta Salad

Ingredients

2 cups Arugula, chopped

1 cup full cream yogurt

½ cup mayonnaise

Two cloves, minced

Three tablespoons extra virgin olive oil

One tablespoon lemon juice, fresh

Two large carrots, grated

Three large tomatoes, sliced

Ten olives pitted and halved

½ cup leeks, chopped

1 cup whole wheat pasta

½ teaspoon black pepper

One medium-sized bell pepper, sliced

½ teaspoon basil

½ teaspoon cilantro

Sea salt

Directions

- Cook the pasta by boiling or following the instructions on the pack.
- Add all the other ingredients to a large bowl and combine well.
- Add the pasta to the other ingredients and toss well to coat thoroughly.
- Serve immediately or refrigerate for a day.

Calais Salmon Salad

Ingredients

3 cups lentils, drained and rinsed

One medium-sized green bell pepper, diced

12-ounce salmon drained and flaked

Five tablespoons extra virgin olive oil

Four tablespoons lemon juice, fresh

Two tablespoons parsley, chopped

2 cups green peas, cleaned

1 cup kale

2 cups spinach

One large white onion, chopped

One large carrot, grated

½ teaspoon chili

Sea salt

Directions

- Combine all the ingredients except the vegetables in a large bowl. Toss well.
- In a separate bowl, add some salt, lemon juice, and olive oil. Mix well then add the vegetables and combine well.
- Serve the greens with a topping of the salmon.

CHAPTER FIVE
Savory

Tuna with Rice and Veggies

Ingredients

1 ½ cup brown rice

Four tablespoons extra virgin olive oil

1 cup turnip, chopped

2 cups broccoli, chopped

2 pounds light tuna,

One onion, sliced

One green bell pepper, sliced

One clove garlic, minced

½ teaspoon basil

½ teaspoon thyme

½ teaspoon curry

½ teaspoon rosemary

½ teaspoon chili

½ teaspoon paprika

One lemon

Sea salt

Directions

- Preheat oven to 375°C.
- Cook the rice by boiling or following the instructions on the pack.
- Add the turnip and broccoli with some oil, salt, and pepper in a bowl. Combine well.
- Arrange the vegetables carefully on a baking sheet and bake for 12 – 15 minutes.
- Cut the lemon into half, then cut the half lemon into four equal sizes. Keep the other half to one side.
- Place the tuna on the baking sheet with the vegetables moved to one side. Sprinkle with the spices, garlic, and onion. Cook for 15 – 20 minutes.
- To a small bowl, add the remaining spices, the other half of the lemon squeezed in. Mix well.

- Portion the rice and top with the vegetables and tuna. Drizzle the lemon mixture and enjoy!

Santorini Salad Nachos

Ingredients

4 cups pita chips

1 cup leek, chopped

Three tablespoons extra virgin olive oil

One clove garlic, crushed

One medium-sized onion, thinly sliced

½ cup hummus

Three tablespoons olives pitted and halved

Two large tomatoes, quartered

1 ½ tablespoon lemon juice, fresh

½ teaspoon black pepper

½ tablespoon oregano

½ teaspoon paprika

½ cup feta cheese, crumbled

Sea salt

Directions

- In a bowl, combine lemon juice, spices, and hummus.
- Lay out the pita chips on a flat surface. Apply the hummus mixture over it. Top with olives, garlic, leek, tomatoes, cheese. Cover with the remaining hummus mixture.

Serve and have fun!

Tuscan Turkey

Ingredients

20 ounces boneless turkey breast, cut into 5

One large red bell pepper, sliced

One small onion, sliced

One clove garlic, crushed

6 cups broccoli

Three tablespoons extra virgin olive oil

One large tomato, chopped

One teaspoon allspice

½ teaspoon jalapeno

4 ounces mozzarella, sliced

Two tablespoons spicy barbecue sauce

Sea salt

Directions

- Spray baking oil on a baking sheet and preheat oven to 295°C.
- Sprinkle turkey with spices and apply barbecue sauce over it generously. Arrange onions, tomatoes over it.
- Arrange the turkey on one side of the baking sheet.
- To a large bowl, add the broccoli, spices, salt, and oil. Combine well and arrange it next to the turkey on the baking sheet.
- Bake for about 25 – 30 minutes.
- Serve warm.

Eggplant Lasagna Rolls

Four large eggplants, trimmed

2 ½ cup crushed tomatoes

Two cloves garlic, minced

One onion, chopped

½ teaspoon jalapeno

3 cups mixed cheese

½ cup hazelnut crushed

Five tablespoons extra virgin olive oil

1 ½ teaspoon Italian seasoning

Sea salt

Directions

- Coat baking sheets or foil with cooking spray and arrange in baking pans.
- Preheat oven to 375°C.
- Cut eggplant lengthwise into ¼ inch thick strips.
- Dowse the eggplant strips with olive oil and some salt.
- Place on the baking sheet and bake for 15 – 20 minutes.
- Remove from the oven and set aside.

- Turn down the heat to 325°C.
- Add the tomatoes, pepper, spices, and onion in a bowl and combine well. Pour the mixture into a baking pan.
- Mix the cheese with some garlic and pepper in a bowl.
- Apply the cheese mixture in the eggplant strips. Fold the slices and place them facing down onto the baking sheets.
- Bake for about 20 minutes.
- Pour the hazelnut, garlic and some salt into a blender. Blender until thoroughly crumbled.
- Sauté in 1 tablespoon olive oil over medium heat in a saucepan for about 2 minutes.
- Top the eggplant with the hazelnut mixture.

Parmesan Risotto Quinoa

Ingredients

1 cup wild rice

2 cups quinoa

Ten tablespoons extra virgin olive oil

Four cloves garlic, crushed

Three tablespoons red wine vinegar

½ teaspoon paprika

½ teaspoon thyme

¼ walnuts, silvered

½ teaspoon black pepper

2 cups Parmesan cheese

½ cup leek

One teaspoon basil

One teaspoon cilantro

Sea salt

Directions

- Preheat oven to 365°C and spray cooking oil on baking sheets.
- Cook the rice following the instructions on the pack and set aside.
- Prepare the quinoa according to

instructions.
- Pour in the walnuts, garlic, and other ingredients into the blender. Blend at high speed until smooth. Add some oil to the mixture and blend for one more minute.
- Heat 4 tablespoons of olive oil in a saucepan over medium heat and add the quinoa and rice. Stir continuously for about 5 minutes. Add the walnut mixture and stir well to combine for about 2 minutes.
- Take off the heat and add the cheese.
- Serve warm with some smoked tuna or chicken.
- Enjoy!

Spicy Couscous with Tuna

Ingredients

2 pounds salmon fillet

Six tablespoons sun-dried tomato

Four tablespoons extra virgin olive oil

½ lemon

1 ½ cup couscous, whole wheat

Two scallions, sliced

½ teaspoon black pepper

2 cups chicken broth

Eight tablespoons olives pitted and halved

Three cloves garlic, crushed

One small onion, sliced

One large carrot, cubed

½ teaspoon paprika

Sea salt

Directions

- Squeeze the lemon on the fillet.
- Sauté the carrots in olive oil over medium heat for 3 minutes. Remove from the saucepan.
- Add the couscous and the scallions to the pan for 2 minutes. Stir continuously.
- Add the olives, broth and other spices.

- Pour in the carrots into the couscous and add the salmon to the mixture. Cook for 10 – 15 minutes.
- Serve warm.

The Essential DASH Diet Cookbook for Beginners

Recipes to Lower Blood Pressure, Lose Weight, Reduce Cholesterol Levels and Boost Metabolism

By

Rina S. Gritton

Acknowledgements

This book could not have been written without the guidance and generosity of many people. To all of you who encouraged and stood by me, thank you.

Copyright © 2019 Rina S. Gritton

The author retains all rights. No part of this document may be reproduced or transmitted in any form or by any means, electronic or mechanical, including photocopying, recording, or by any information storage and retrieval system without permission in writing from the author. The unauthorized reproduction or distribution of this copyrighted work is illegal.

Disclaimer

The information contained in this material is based on years of several types of research by scientists, dieticians and other professionals in the health field. Whatever you read within the pages of this book is for purely of informational purposes only and is not to be taken as a guide for diagnosis for any psychological or medical condition, nor to treat, mitigate or prevent any disease. Do not discard the professional advice from qualified health care personnel based on the information you get from this book. This book is not intended to be, and you should decide your health based on appropriate discussions with a qualified medical doctor or healthcare professional.

Introduction

High blood pressure also commonly referred to as hypertension is becoming prevalent in our societies at this age and time. It is the drastically reduces the life expectancy rates of individuals who have the unfortunate luck of coming down with it. Folks with higher blood pressures are more likely to have shorter life spans. Due to its nature, it may go unnoticed and untreated leading to severe conditions such as kidney malfunctioning, heart failure, stroke, etc. The causes of hypertension can be linked to a host of factors which include and are not limited to lifestyle habits and dietary factors.

Due to this disease not been noticed and managed on time, it kills in the most silent of ways and can bring about a reduced and unwholesome quality of life with complications that leaves one going in and out of the ER pumped full of medications all the time. In a healthy individual, there is a regular flow of blood flowing from the arteries to all significant organs delivering life-sustaining oxygen and essential nutrients. When there is a restriction of this flow due to clogged arteries or other conditions, the flow of blood becomes forced leading to an increase in the pressure and eventual damage of essential organs in the body. A healthy weight loss can significantly bring blood pressure levels to normal levels and most medications that are considered "normal" like most pain killers, OTC prescriptions can elevate blood pressure levels.

The Wrong Move

Most methods and approaches to treating and mitigating hypertension can be described as been harmful and can potentially bring about severe health challenges. So instead of going down the well-known route with the consumption and constant intake of medications to treat the condition, you need to understand what high blood pressure is. I have had discussions with people who say that the situation is in their genetic makeup and that is a wrong assumption. How you live your life conditions and impacts your DNA and may or may not predispose you to the condition. How active you are, your nutritional choices, how you process daily life struggles, the presence of chemicals and pollutants all around.

It is a common practice to make use of anti-hypertensive medications to lower high blood pressure, but these prescriptions hardly ever do the job. The condition is most times not adequately brought under control by only sticking to, and only a handful out of numerous folks suffering from the condition have it under control.

A New Way

We have become fixated to treating high blood pressure with medications which I will say is rather easy and most times ineffective while we ignore the natural and wholesome way through the consumption of appropriate foods. When you eat foods that contain the right amount of nutrients that will keep your blood pressure healthy, you will be kept away from medications that can be prohibitively expensive and have some adverse side effects too. The type of life that you live can also bring about an increase in blood pressure levels, and stress levels hormones mostly cause this. This is most times that event that brings about a chain reaction that ultimately brings about the dreaded heart attack.

You should know that there are quite a lot of natural foods that will get your blood flowing without the chemicals that may do more harm than good. Dietary food habits such as sticking to a flexitarian or whole food diet, adding supplements, controlling your stress levels are very important in keeping an optimum body weight. A healthy body weight is essential in maintaining and keeping your blood levels regular. It is also pertinent to know that adopting a healthy lifestyle keeps your insulin levels under check as a high level of this hormone may likely have effects on other processes within the body such as increased weight gain, clogged blood vessels, high blood pressure, etc. Such persons are likely to come down with a stroke, heart attack and other diseases which are as a result of clogged blood vessels.

Salt

The moment high blood pressure is talked about, that particular conversation will be incomplete without a mention about salt. A few decades ago, salt was a store of value and highly precious used sparingly, but nowadays, it is as common as the very air that we breathe. That's the inherent problem of this very valuable substance that adds taste and flavor to our dishes. The relationship between hypertension and salt is irrefutable in a segment of the population that is predisposed to the effects of salt on their blood pressures. Don't get the picture wrong here; salt is necessary for the general wellbeing of the human body as the sodium content is vital in relation to other ions such as potassium for the proper functioning of the body system. When there is a disproportionate level of either ion in the system over some time, the body goes into a downward spiral with essential organs failing due to an increased or drastic drop in blood pressure. In essence, there needs to be a balanced intake of both ions and other micro-ions for a healthy functional body.

So how do you get your daily intake of potassium? Simple! Get adequate amounts of bananas, vegetables, fruits such as avocados, and pawpaw. As with everything that has to do with your health and blood pressure, you should consume moderation to avoid overloading on any one nutrient or ion.

The knee jerk reactionary treatment once one is diagnosed with a high blood pressure condition is to reduce the amount of salt intake immediately. This action is unhealthy, and there have been reports of individuals who are on low salt diets who died compared to those who did not cut back on their sodium intake. The loophole to be used here is to take a wide berth around highly processed foods that mostly contain a high amount of refined salts and focus more on the consumption of whole natural foods that have undergone little or no processing. Whole natural food also contains sodium as in the highly processed ones, but the significant difference is that in the natural state and pure with no artificial additives.

The recommended daily allowance of salt for the average human is about 2200 milligrams. You can get your daily dose in some of these foods; beans, meat, vegetables, etc. It will be almost impossible for some folks to cook without making use of a pinch of salt for taste and flavoring. In this case, it will be best to make use of salts that have not undergone any refining, and that is still in its natural state, e.g. sea or kosher salt, Himalayan salt as long as your meal is balanced and has enough potassium to balance the amount of sodium you are taking in at any given time. For those who make use of strong spices with incredible flavors, there will be no need to add much salt to your dishes. Another way to add salt to your cooking is to add a pinch to your plate after your cooking. You will get the best taste out of your meals this way.

This does not give you the free card to eat salt by the boatload as you can cause severe irreversible damage to your system if you go down this route. Salt is not bad for you as we have been meant to believe. That salt that you eat day in day out in all that highly refined and processed foods that we have on shelves in the supermarkets are the poisons that are causing mortal harm to we humans. The big food companies continually add salts to all classes of their food products, and they are empty in that there are no health benefits to be derived from these "salts." These salts are an illusion to our taste buds as they deceive our tongues from tasting the poisons that are the ingredients used in making the packaged deaths that we ignorantly embrace.

We have also been made to believe that the so-called iodized salt is good for us. That is a blatant lie that aims to put more money into the pockets of the fat cats. Iodized salt merely is salt that has undergone a lot of refining then having iodine added to it to prevent goiter supposedly. The truth is that if you eat enough wholesome meals such as seafood (crab, prawn, fish, etc), then there will be no need to add a form of these so-called iodized salts to your dishes! Though there is a possibility of an individual coming down with a thyroid problem if there is not enough iodine in the diet, so too if one is taking in excess iodine. To avoid this problem, it is best you stick to the natural forms of salts that have not been refined in any way and also try to focus more on dishes that contain natural forms of iodine.

Dietary Recommendations

To get your blood pressure levels under control, the first step to take is to embrace a healthy eating habit. Whole food diets will provide your body with all the essential nutrients that are needed to start the healing process. Once you begin to cut out those harmful "food" substances, you will start to feel much better with the elimination of those addictive substances. Your blood pressure will adjust to its average level within a few days. Food is an excellent healer and can be therapeutic and also cause grievous harm if misused. With this most important fact, you should leverage the fantastic healing properties of wholesome food. So how can you harness these powers that food has to reduce your dangerously high blood levels? Follow these simple steps;

Cut out the sugars; diets full of empty sugars, highly refined carbohydrates, when taken into the human system, brings about a spike in the insulin levels which is a precursor to insulin resistance and finally type 2 diabetes. When this condition persists for a long while, it invariably leads to hypertension, low libido, propensity to cancer and other deleterious health effects. To avoid all these health conditions or manage it, cut back on the amount of sugar in whatever form that you take in.

Have a healthy combination of vegetables, protein, and fat for breakfast. These are an excellent food combination to kick start your system any day.

Ensure that you restrict your alcohol intake as making it a habit might lead to an increase in blood pressure levels and other side effects. Regular consumption of alcohol creates a skewed sugar level in the blood and also negatively affects the triglycerides levels and functions in the body.

Your dinner should be had at least three hours before you sleep.

Focus on wholesome plant diets that are rich in potassium and other essential nutrients. These are mostly vegetables, fruits, seeds having high fiber contents and nuts. The principal function of potassium on the human body is that it counters the effects of sodium. It aids in the relaxation of the blood vessels which invariably means that the blood pressure levels are reduced. The majority of people only consume about half the recommended daily allowance of this mineral. Ensure you try to up the amount of potassium you consume daily to at least 4,500mg daily through a lot of vegetables and fruits. Vegetables are rich in phytonutrients, anti-inflammatory substances, and antioxidants that are essential in maintaining optimal health levels.

Make sure that you eat good fat daily, and these can be found in olive oil, coconut butter, seeds and nuts, organic eggs, milk, beef and seafood with relatively large amounts of oil, e.g. herring, sardines, salmon, etc.

Water is life, and it cannot be overemphasized; drink at least eight glasses of clean, pure water daily and these amounts may increase if the weather is hot or if you are engaged in strenuous activities.

Incorporate a reasonably decent size of protein into your meals daily.

Do I need to tell you to avoid junk foods?

Fill your kitchen shelves with real wholesome foods that cuts down on your chances of coming down with diabetes, enhances the functioning of your liver, regulates your blood sugar levels and so much more. Unprocessed foods improve the metabolism of the body, and a disease that comes with the onset of aging is also drastically reduced.

Fats that are contained in a lot of baked goods and highly processed foods should be strictly avoided.

Physical Activity; Engaging in moderate to intense physical activities/ exercise regularly throughout a week strengthens your muscles, heart and other organs. Your heart will require less energy and force to move blood through the vessels, and thus less pressure is generated. Exercising is also very good for you if you intend to get rid of that excess body weight, have a high level of mental alertness, increased libido and cut down on the amount of cholesterol in your body.

Exercising strengthens the muscles and this result in a reduction of mostly unwanted body fat. The cardiovascular regime to be carried out at least four times a week for 20 – 30 minutes goes a long way in ensuring you do not come down with any sudden heart problems. You may be of the school of thought who see those exercising as been overly conscious of their body or who have got a lot of time on their hands. This is a very wrong notion as exercising is a must for everyone though the intensity and frequency may be slightly different for all individuals due to body type and other activities which may take up your time. Constant physical activities cut down the risk of coming down with a lot of ailments such as osteoarthritis, dementia, diabetes, cardio issues, obesity, etc. Our bodies are designed to be in perpetual motion, and if you live a sedentary lifestyle, you will be likely to have a lot of health issues in your old age.

Sleep is a time when your body gets to rest and regenerate tissues and cells. With the active lifestyles we are currently living, it is almost impossible to get the required number of hours of sleep that we need daily. To ensure that you sleep as soon as you get into bed, cut down on stimulating activities about one to two hours before you sleep. This can take a while before your body adapts to it as it is already used to that rhythm which needs to be broken to develop a healthier one. For example, ensure that you maintain a regular sleeping time and stick to it and make use of your bed for sleep and possibly sex only. Do not eat, read, go through your phone or watch television in bed. Those are all terrible bed habits. When the night time comes, and you hit the bed, turn off all the lights, shut the curtain and remove all forms of distractions that may interfere with your sleep. A dark, serene room is a prerequisite for having a good night rest and healthy life.

Starting with the DASH Diet

The DASH diet is quite easy to start and maintain as it does not involve any special skills or foods. All you must to do is keep a healthy eating habit with meals from all the major food classes and achieving your recommended daily allowance of calories. The amount of calories you are permitted to consume each day is determined by your health status, sex, age, activity levels, weight, etc. If your primary goal is to add some muscle mass and add some more weight, then your calorie intake will invariably have to increase.

Take a look at what your eating pattern was like before you decided to start with the DASH diet. Reduce the servings, cut out unhealthy foods, junks, sugars, and empty foods. Reduce your refined salt intake and try as much as you can to not put the salt shaker anywhere around the dining table. Spice up your meals with natural herbs and spices

As with any process, change is always a bit hard to adapt to. In trying to eat healthily, ensure that it is a gradual process over days and weeks. Give your taste buds some time to get used to the new dietary intakes. Increase your vegetable and fruit consumption, cut down on the alcohol. Take more of whole wheat products and less red meat. Eat more seafood and less refined sugar.

As you change your diet, there is also the need to make wise and healthy changes to your lifestyle. For example, if you are a bit overweight and you aim to shed some fat, get some wholesome food with relatively low-calorie contents and increase your physical activities. This should not be a sudden act; it should be done slowly to give your body the ability to adapt to the change. However, before you start with a weight loss program using DASH diets or any other form of menus, talk to your doctor for professional advice. The DASH diet has so many benefits from reducing your risks of coming down with cardiovascular problems to losing weight and generally providing your body with the very much needed healthy nutrients.

Chapter One

Prawn and Green Salad

Ingredients

2 pounds fresh prawns, peeled and deveined

1 cup kale, chopped

1 cup spinach, chopped

1 cup eggplant, thinly sliced

Two tablespoons extra virgin olive oil

Two large tomatoes, sliced

One large white onion, thinly sliced

Two cloves garlic, minced

One tablespoon honey

3 cups green salad greens

2 cups yellow, frozen con

One teaspoon black pepper

Two tablespoons canola oil

One teaspoon Dijon mustard

One teaspoon parsley

One teaspoon lemon zest

Sea salt

Directions

- Add the mustard, vinegar, and honey to a bowl. Combine well.
- Put a large saucepan on medium heat.
- Introduce some olive oil and stir fry the corn for about 2 – 3 minutes.
- Add the cleaned prawns to a large bowl and drizzle some salt and pepper over it.
- Add the prawn to the saucepan with some olive oil and cook for about 4 – 5 minutes. Add the corn and stir for another 1 minute.
- Add all the salad ingredients to another large bowl. Toss properly to combine.

Serve the salad and the stir-fried prawns immediately.

- Enjoy.

Veal with Spicy Tomato Curry

Ingredients

Eight boneless veal

6 cups brown rice, cooked

Two large apples, thinly sliced

One large red onion, chopped

Two cloves garlic, minced

Six tablespoons butter, divided

Two tablespoons sugar

One teaspoon chili

One teaspoon oregano

½ teaspoon curry

½ teaspoon thyme

Sea salt

Directions

- Add three tablespoons of the butter to a large skillet over medium heat. Brown the veal for about 3 minutes on each side.
- Add the remaining butter to the same skillet over medium heat and sauté the garlic and onions for about 1 – 2 minutes. Add all the other ingredients and spices.
- Put back the veal to the skillet and allow the mixture to simmer for 6 – 8 minutes.
- Remove it from the cooker and keep in a cool area for about 4 – 6 minutes.
- Serve warm with rice.

Crunchy Overnight Oats

Ingredients

1 cup slivered almonds

½ cup thinly chopped apples

1 cup old-fashioned oats

Two tablespoons honey

One tablespoon chia seeds

½ cup mixed berries

½ cup of coconut milk

½ cup Greek yogurt

Directions

- Add all the ingredients for the oats in a large bowl.
- Pour the mixture into a mason jar.
- Seal very tight and set in the fridge overnight.
- Serve cold or warm slightly for about 2 minutes in a large pan.
- Serve immediately.

Bangkok Chicken Macaroni

Ingredients

4 cups, shredded cooked chicken

1 cup carrots, thinly sliced

1 cup green peas

One large onion thinly sliced

Two cloves garlic, minced

Three tablespoons extra virgin olive oil

One pack whole wheat macaroni

Two large tomatoes, sliced

One teaspoon basil

One teaspoon soy sauce

½ cup peanut sauce

1 cup eggplant, sliced

Directions

- Prepare the macaroni following instructions on the pack.
- To a large saucepan, pour the olive oil and sauté the onions, garlic, green peas, and carrot for about 4 – 6 minutes.

- Add the peanut sauce, spices, chicken and the macaroni.
- Toss and cook for another 2 minutes.
- Serve warm.

Bacon - Stuffed Eggplant

Ingredients

Eight medium-sized eggplants

1 ½ pound smoked bacon

½ cup mixed cheese

One medium onion, thinly sliced

Three cloves garlic, minced

One large tomato, sliced

One large green bell pepper, deseeded and sliced

One teaspoon oregano

One teaspoon parsley

One teaspoon black pepper

One teaspoon cilantro

1 ½ cup bread crumbs

Two tablespoons extra virgin olive oil

Sea salt

Directions

- Preheat oven to 290°C.
- Cut the eggplant vertically in half. Take most of the pulp and diced the removed flesh.
- Put the eggplants in oven-safe bowls, seal it and microwave for about 3 – 4 minutes.
- Add some olive oil to a large saucepan. Over medium heat, steam the pork and eggplant pulp for 8 – 10 minutes. Add the onions, garlic, and other spices.
- Fill the eggplant with the bacon mixture.
- Place the eggplant in baking dishes, cover and bake for 18 – 20 minutes.

- Apply the cheese over the eggplant and remove the cover while you bake for another 3 – 5 minutes.
- Serve warm.
- Enjoy.

Spicy Brown Beans Hummus

Ingredients

3 cups cooked brown beans

One large onion, sliced

Three cloves garlic, minced

One teaspoon jalapeno

Two tablespoons cilantro, fresh

One teaspoon curry

Two tablespoons lemon juice

Four tablespoons tahini

2 cups of mixed vegetables

Sea salt

Directions

- Place the beans and other ingredients into a high powered blender.
- Blitz at high speed until a smooth consistency is obtained.
- Pour the contents into a container and add the cilantro.
- Serve with whole wheat bread or tacos.
- Refrigerate to preserve.

Peppered Spicy Walnuts

Ingredients

3 cups walnuts

½ teaspoon nutmeg

½ teaspoon paprika

One teaspoon chili

½ teaspoon garlic powder

½ teaspoon ginger powder

½ teaspoon cinnamon

½ teaspoon coriander

Sea salt

One tablespoon extra virgin olive oil

Directions

- Combine the spices in a bowl.
- To another separate bowl, combine the walnuts and the olive oil.
- Sprinkle the walnut with the spices and toss well.
- Pour the spiced walnuts onto a greased baking foil.
- Bake at 290°C for 18 – 20 minutes and stir intermittently.
- Allow to air cool then transfer to an airtight mason jar.

Black Bean Tomato Soup

Ingredients

2 cups carrots, chopped

Two large onions, thinly sliced

3 cups brown beans, parboiled

8 cups vegetable broth

Three cloves garlic, minced

1 cup cilantro, fresh

One teaspoon ginger powder

One teaspoon oregano

Two large tomatoes, chopped

One teaspoon jalapeno

Four tablespoons extra virgin olive oil

Sea salt

Directions

- Sauté onions, garlic, and carrots in olive oil over medium heat for 4 – 6 minutes.
- Add the broth, spices and the beans and bring to boil.
- Allow simmering for about 15 minutes.

- Add the cilantro and tomatoes, salt and stir.
- Let it simmer for 2 - 3 minutes.
- Serve warm.

Spicy Grilled Tuna

Ingredients

2 pounds tuna fillet

Two tablespoons extra virgin olive oil

One teaspoon jalapeno

1 ½ tablespoon soy sauce

½ tablespoon brown sugar

½ teaspoon garlic powder

One teaspoon allspice

One teaspoon mustard, ground

½ teaspoon dill weed

½ teaspoon oregano

Sea salt

Directions

- Combine all the ingredients except for the tuna in a bowl.
- Brush the tuna fillet with the spices.
- Place the tuna with the skin down on a greased baking sheet and cover it with another foil.
- Grill over medium heat for about 12 – 15 minutes.
- Serve warm with vegetable salad.

Zesty Peppered Chicken

Ingredients

Two tablespoons extra virgin olive oil

½ teaspoon paprika

Six chicken breasts, boneless

Three cloves garlic, minced

1 cup carrots, minced

One large red onion, thinly sliced

Two teaspoons lemon zest

One teaspoon black pepper

One teaspoon chili

½ teaspoon oregano

One large tomato, quartered

One medium-sized yellow bell pepper, sliced

Sea salt

Directions

- Add the olive oil to a large saucepan over medium heat. Sauté the carrots, onions, and garlic for 2 minutes. Add the other spices and stir.
- Place the chicken breasts over the carrots.
- Cover the pan and cook for 15 – 20 minutes.
- Serve warm and enjoy.

Chapter Two

Crispy Rainbow Salad

Ingredients

2 cups carrots, chopped

One large cucumber, thinly sliced

2 cups kale, chopped

One large tomato, thinly sliced

1 cup cilantro

2 cups snap peas

2 cups romaine lettuce, chopped

Directions

- Add all the vegetables to a bowl and toss well to combine.
- Put in a fridge to chill.
- Serve with salad dressing of your choice.

Cucumber Tomato Gazpacho

Ingredients

One large cucumber, minced

Three large heirloom tomatoes, diced

Three tablespoons olive oil

3 cups vegetable juice

One large red onion, chopped

Four cloves garlic, minced

One large red bell pepper, sliced

One tablespoon apple cider vinegar

One teaspoon parsley

One teaspoon black pepper

One teaspoon basil

Sea salt

Directions

- Add the ingredients to a large bowl.
- Combine well.

- Put into a refrigerator for about 30 minutes.
- Serve chilled.

Garlic Hummus Dip

Ingredients

3 cups brown beans, cooked

Four cloves garlic, minced

One large white onion, chopped

One large tomato, chopped

One teaspoon curry

One teaspoon turmeric

One teaspoon ginger, grated

One teaspoon paprika

½ teaspoon cumin

One teaspoon black pepper

Two tablespoons extra virgin olive oil

Sea salt

Directions

- Sauté onions, garlic, and tomato for 2 minutes in olive oil over medium heat.
- Add the other spices and allow cooking for a further 5 minutes.
- Pour in the beans and cook for 3 minutes. Stir intermittently.
- Pour the contents into a high powered food processor and blend until smooth.
- Serve warm with pita or tacos.
- Enjoy!

Grilled Kale Lentils Creamy Dip

Ingredients

4 cups kale, chopped

3 cups lentils

1 cup Greek yogurt

2 cloves, garlic

One medium-sized yellow onion, chopped

One teaspoon black pepper

Sea salt

Directions

- Preheat oven to 280°C.
- Add the vegetables and other ingredients with to a bowl and combine well.
- Pour the contents of the bowl into a casserole dish.
- Bake for 22 – 24 minutes.
- Serve with pita bread or whole wheat bread and enjoy.

Ginger Marinated Pork Chops

Ingredients

2 pounds boneless pork chops

One teaspoon jalapeno

One tablespoon ginger, grated

Two cloves garlic, minced

One teaspoon oregano

Two teaspoon lime juice

One teaspoon paprika

Sea salt

Directions

- Set the pork chops into a bowl.
- Add the spices and other ingredients.
- Using your hands, thoroughly work the spices into the pork.
- Allow the pork to marinate for 45 – 60 minutes.
- Grill the pork on high heat for about 6 – 8 minutes on each side.
- Serve with salad, some hummus, and rice with some cold fresh juice to go with it.

Chicken Sausage with Sweet Potatoes

Ingredients

1 pound cooked chicken sausage

One large white onion, sliced

Two cloves garlic, minced

½ teaspoon curry

½ teaspoon thyme

Four tablespoons extra virgin olive oil

½ teaspoon black pepper

1 pound sweet potatoes, cleaned, peeled and cubed

One large tomato, sliced

1 cup carrot, grated

½ cup green peas

½ teaspoon oregano

Sea salt

Directions

- Add olive oil to a skillet and gently heat over medium heat.

- Sauté the onion, garlic, and potatoes for about 10 – 12 minutes. Put in the peppers and spices and continue to stir.
- Pour in the chicken sausage and stir. Allow cooking for another 8 – 10 minutes.
- Add the carrots, tomatoes and green peas and stir. Cook for 2 – 4 minutes.
- Serve warm.

Spag Veggie Soup

Ingredients

4 cups vegetable broth

Three tablespoons extra virgin olive oil

One onion, sliced

Four cloves garlic, minced

2 cups carrots, chopped

1 cup kale, chopped

1 cup zucchini, thinly sliced

3 cups of water

One teaspoon parsley

½ teaspoon cumin

One pack spaghetti

Directions

- Sauté the vegetables in olive oil over medium heat for 5 minutes in a large pot.
- Pour in the water and broth and allow to boil.
- Introduce the spaghetti and cook until it is well prepared.
- Serve with some cheese toppings.

Quinoa Burgers

2 cups quinoa

1 cup shallots, finely chopped

Two cloves garlic

One teaspoon black pepper

½ cup parsley, finely chopped

Three eggs, beaten

½ cup carrot, grated

¼ cup whole wheat flour

½ teaspoon paprika

One green bell pepper, sliced

One tomato, sliced

Three tablespoons extra virgin olive oil

Sea salt

Directions

- Add the quinoa and the other ingredients except the olive oil in a large bowl.
- Combine thoroughly making use of your hands.
- Add olive oil into a skillet and cook the quinoa patties over medium heat, 4 – 6 minutes per side.

Grilled Sirloin Beef with Vegetables

Ingredients

2 pounds beef

One large zucchini

2 cups spinach, chopped

1 cup Brussels sprouts

Four cloves garlic, chopped

Two tablespoons extra virgin olive oil

Four large heirloom tomatoes, quartered

½ teaspoon rosemary

½ teaspoon sage

One teaspoon ginger, grated

One tablespoon apple cider vinegar

One teaspoon lemon zest

½ teaspoon oregano

One teaspoon basil

One teaspoon black pepper

Sea salt

Directions

- To prepare the marinade, combine all the spices, vinegar, zest, olive oil, and salt.
- Combine the beef and some of the marinade in a bowl.
- Pour the marinated beef into a Ziploc bag and keep in a fridge for 60 – 90 minutes.
- Cover a baking sheet with some foil and grease.
- Place the tomatoes, sprouts, and zucchini on the foil.
- Remove the beef out of the bag and grill over medium to high heat, 10 – 12 minutes per side. Take it off the heat and cover.
- Grill the vegetables for about 2 – 3 minutes per side.
- Add some the remaining marinade to the vegetables and toss.

- Serve the vegetables with the grilled beef.
- Enjoy!

Chapter Three

Pasta and Shrimp with Sautéed Vegetables

Ingredients

2 cups pasta, uncooked

Three cloves garlic, minced

2 pounds shrimp, peeled and deveined

One large onion, sliced

One medium-sized green bell pepper, sliced

Three tablespoons extra virgin olive oil

½ cup eggplant, sliced

1 cup lentils

½ cup carrot, grated

One teaspoon jalapeno

1 cup mixed cheese

One tablespoon lemon juice

½ teaspoon basil

½ teaspoon oregano

One tablespoon cilantro

Sea salt

Directions

- Prepare your pasta by going with the instructions on the pack.
- To a large saucepan, add the olive oil and sauté the vegetables over medium heat.
- Add the lemon juice and shrimp. Stir well and add the spices. Cook for 5 – 7 minutes on low heat.
- Take the pasta off the heat and add the cheese.
- Serve warm.

Spicy Grilled Salmon

Ingredients

Eight salmon fillets

One small onion, chopped

Two cloves garlic, minced

½ teaspoon chili

½ cup green bell pepper, chopped

One tablespoon extra virgin olive oil

½ cup fresh parsley

½ teaspoon curry

Sea salt

Directions

- Combine all your ingredients except for the fish in a bowl.
- Drizzle the spice over the salmon fillets.
- Place the fish over a grill at medium heat and cook on each side for about 3 – 4 minutes.
- Serve warm with some salad.

Cocoa Smoothie with Banana

Ingredients

4 cups full cream coconut milk

Two large bananas, peeled

½ cup of cocoa powder

One tablespoon flax seed

Ice cubes

Directions

- Pour in all the ingredients into a high powered blender.
- Blitz at high speed until smooth.
- Serve chilled.

Peanut and Berry Mix

Ingredients

2 cups frozen mixed berries

1 cup roasted peanuts

½ cup coconut, shredded

½ cup mango

2 cups Greek yogurt

Ice cubes

Directions

- Combine all the ingredients into a blender.
- Blend at high speed until a creamy consistency is obtained.
- Serve chilled.

Chicken Salad and Kale Sandwiches

Ingredients

1 pound boneless chicken breast, smoked

1 cup shallot, chopped

Four tablespoons lemon juice

Three tablespoons extra virgin olive oil

One small zucchini, peeled, seeded and diced

One teaspoon cayenne

One clove garlic, minced

Ten slices whole wheat bread

One teaspoon dill

1 cup kale, chopped

Sea salt

Directions

- Combine the chicken, shallots onions and other ingredients in a large bowl.
- Scoop the chicken mixture onto one slice of bread and cover with another slice of bread.
- Press down the sandwich firmly.
- Pack in your lunch box or enjoy immediately!

Roasted Brussels Sprouts

Ingredients

1 pound Brussels sprouts

Five cloves garlic, minced

½ teaspoon black pepper

½ teaspoon ginger powder

½ teaspoon rosemary

Four tablespoons extra virgin olive oil

½ teaspoon cayenne pepper

Sea salt

Directions

- Preheat the oven to 320°C.
- Cover a baking sheet with a foil.
- Combine the sprouts and three tablespoons of olive oil.
- Add the black pepper and some salt.
- Pour in the sprouts onto the baking sheet and bake for 14 – 16 minutes.
- Pour in cayenne pepper and some olive oil into a bowl with the other spices. Combine well.

- Drizzle the olive oil mixture over the roasted sprouts. Toss to combine well.
- Bake for another 6 – 8 minutes.
- Serve immediately.

Creamy Mashed Potatoes

Ingredients

3 pounds potatoes, peeled and cubed

½ cup extra virgin olive oil

1 cup mixed cheese

½ cup cream

Four cloves garlic, minced

One large onion, thinly sliced

One large red bell pepper

One teaspoon basil

½ teaspoon oregano

One teaspoon black pepper

Sea salt

Directions

- Cover the potatoes, onions, and garlic with water in a pot.
- Allow the contents of the pot to boil, and then allow simmering for 20 – 24 minutes.
- Take it from the heat and then drain the water into a bowl.
- Add the cream, olive oil, cheese and some of the water from the cooked potatoes to the pot.
- Thoroughly mash the potatoes using any suitable kitchen utensil.
- Serve warm with a side of salad.

Cancun Quinoa

Ingredients

1 ½ cup quinoa, rinsed

One medium eggplant, chopped

1 cup mixed cheese

Three cloves garlic, minced

Two tablespoons extra virgin olive oil

1 cup brown beans, drained

One tablespoon cilantro

2 ¼ cups water

One teaspoon paprika

½ teaspoon oregano

One teaspoon jalapeno

Sea salt

Directions

- Heat oil over low to medium heat in a skillet.
- Pour in the quinoa, onions, and garlic. Stir fry for about 3 – 5 minutes.
- Add in the eggplant and water and heat until it starts boiling.

- Lower the heat and allow to simmering 10 – 12 minutes.
- Add in the spices, cheese, beans, and other ingredients. Mix well and let simmering for another 2 – 3 minutes.
- Serve hot.

Peppered Veal Kabobs

Ingredients

Two large white onions, chopped

One large red bell pepper, seeded and chopped

One tablespoon parsley

One tablespoon cilantro

One tablespoon lime juice

1 pound veal, cubed

One teaspoon black pepper

One small pineapple, cubed

Four large heirloom tomatoes, quartered

Directions

- Add the first ingredients to a bowl, mix well and keep.
- Sprinkle some salt and pepper over the veal and skewer alternately the veal, pineapple, and tomatoes.
- Grill the veal over medium heat for about 12 – 15 minutes while turning it regularly.
- Serve with the salsa.

Turkey Lettuce Wraps

Ingredients

1 pound boneless turkey breasts, cubed

Three tablespoons extra virgin olive oil

Three cloves garlic, minced

One small onion, chopped

½ teaspoon cayenne pepper

One tablespoon teriyaki sauce

Two tablespoons apple cider vinegar

Ten romaine lettuce leaves

One teaspoon ginger, grated

½ cup carrots, grated

½ teaspoon oregano

½ teaspoon soy sauce

¼ cup walnuts, coarsely crushed

Sea salt

Directions

- Add some salt, pepper, garlic, and ginger to the turkey and coat well.
- Add the olive oil to a large saucepan over medium heat. Introduce the turkey and stir fry for about 4 – 6 minutes.
- Take the pan away from the heat and add the walnuts, onions, and carrots. Stir well and allow to sit.

- To a bowl, introduce the remaining ingredients and combine. Pour it over the turkey mixture.
- Scoop the turkey mixture onto the lettuce leaves and seal.
- Serve immediately.

Spinach Beans Sauté with Pasta

Ingredients

4 cups baby spinach, chopped

2 cups brown beans, drained

1 cup white beans, drained

2 cups chicken broth

½ teaspoon black pepper

Five tablespoons extra virgin olive oil

Five cloves garlic, minced

One medium-sized yellow bell pepper, sliced

One tablespoon apple cider vinegar

One large onion, thinly sliced

One pack whole wheat pasta

One teaspoon black pepper

One teaspoon basil

Sea salt

Directions

- Drain all the beans and pour into a bowl. Add some olive oil, black pepper, and salt. Combine well.
- Add some olive oil to a skillet and sauté the onions and garlic for 2 minutes over medium heat.
- Add the broth, beans, and spices. Increase the heat and cook for 5 – 7 minutes.
- Remove the pan from the heat and introduce the vinegar and spinach. Stir well.
- Serve beans immediately with already prepared pasta.

Trout Stuffed Avocado

1 pound trout fillet, smoked

Three tablespoons extra virgin olive oil

One teaspoon black pepper

½ teaspoon paprika

½ teaspoon sage

One clove garlic, crushed

One small onion, thinly sliced

Three avocados, sliced in half

One tablespoon parsley

Two tablespoons lemon juice

Sea salt

Directions

- Add the trout and other ingredients to a large bowl.
- Combine well-making use of your hands.

- Use a spoon to fill each avocado with the trout mixture.
- Enjoy!

Chicken Burger

Ingredients

1 pound ground chicken

Two cloves garlic, minced

One red onion, chopped

Two tablespoons extra virgin olive oil

One teaspoon rosemary

½ teaspoon thyme

One teaspoon jalapeno

½ cup carrot, grated

Sea salt

Directions

- Pour the ground chicken into a bowl and add all the other ingredients.
- Combine the mixture well-making use of your hands.
- Form burger patties with the mixture and grill over medium heat for about 7 – 10 minutes or until well done.
- Place the grilled chicken in between whole wheat bread.

Brown Rice with Vegetable Stir Fry

Ingredients

1 cup shallot, chopped

1 cup carrots, grated

Two large tomatoes, sliced

Three cloves garlic, minced

One large onion, thinly sliced

1 cup green peas

2 cups brown rice, cooked

One teaspoon ginger powder

½ cup roasted almonds, crushed

1 cup broccoli, chopped

One tablespoon flax seeds

Three tablespoons extra virgin olive oil

One teaspoon soy sauce

1 ½ tablespoon apple cider vinegar

One teaspoon black pepper

One teaspoon basil

Two tablespoons fish sauce

½ teaspoon turmeric

Directions

- Add the ginger, vinegar, soy sauce, fish sauce, the spices and some of the olive oil to a small bowl. Combine well.

- Add some olive oil to a skillet over medium heat and sauté the vegetables for about 6 – 10 minutes. Stir continuously.
- Add in the rice, almonds, and sauce and mix properly.
- Cook for another 1 minute.
- Serve immediately.

Chapter Four

Chicken and Quinoa Vegetable Soup

Ingredients

Two large tomatoes, chopped

Three tablespoons extra virgin olive oil

1 cup quinoa

1 cup kale

5 cups vegetable broth

Two cloves garlic, minced

1 cup shallot, chopped

1 cup broccoli, chopped

1 pound chicken breast, cubed and cooked

One teaspoon chili

1 cup spinach, chopped

½ teaspoon sage

½ teaspoon rosemary

One small green bell pepper, thinly sliced

½ teaspoon cumin

Sea salt

Directions

- Pour olive oil into a skillet over low to medium heat.
- Sauté the shallots and garlic for 2 – 3 minutes.
- Add in the quinoa and broth. Allow boiling then reduce to low heat. Add the spices, chicken and other vegetables. Cook for 12 – 15 minutes.
- Serve warm and enjoy!

Grilled Texan Pork Salad

Ingredients

1 pound lean pork

One large yellow bell pepper, sliced

Two tablespoons extra virgin olive oil

2 cups black-eyed peas, cooked

One large tomato

½ teaspoon parsley

½ teaspoon jalapeno

Four large ears corn, cleaned

½ teaspoon garlic powder

Dressing

Four tablespoons lime juice

½ teaspoon chili

½ cup cilantro

One teaspoon basil

Two tablespoons extra virgin olive oil

½ teaspoon oregano

½ teaspoon curry

Sea salt

Directions

- Put the pork into a bowl and sprinkle some salt, pepper, garlic, and other spices over it. Mix it well using your hand.
- Sprinkle some of the oil and spices over the corn, bell pepper, and onions too.
- Place the pork over a grill and heat over medium heat for 10 – 15 minutes on each side or it is done to your desired taste.
- Place the corn, pepper, and onions on the grill too. Cook for 7 – 10 minutes. Turn intermittently.
- Add all the ingredients meant for the dressing into a bowl and whisk well.
- Put the corn and grilled chopped vegetables into a bowl and pour the dressings over it.
- Introduce the cubed pork into the mixture too.

- Add the beans to the salad mixture and toss properly.
- Serve and enjoy.

Quinoa Salad

One pack mixed vegetables

2 cups quinoa, cooked

One large onion, thinly sliced

One clove garlic, chopped

One teaspoon jalapeno

1 cup brown beans, cooked

1 cup mixed cheese

One teaspoon paprika

½ teaspoon basil

½ cup frozen yellow corn

½ cup carrot, chopped

One teaspoon parsley

½ teaspoon cumin

Three tablespoons extra virgin olive oil

Sea salt

Directions

- Gently heat olive oil on low to medium heat in a saucepan.
- Sauté the carrot, onion, garlic, and corn for about 3 minutes. Add the other spices and cook for another 2 minutes.
- Add the quinoa, beans and mixed vegetables. Stir continuously and cook for another 2 minutes.
- Serve with sprinkled cheese.

Vegetable Turkey Soup

Ingredients

2 pounds ground turkey

1 cup kale, chopped

Four cloves garlic, minced

One large onion, thinly sliced

1 cup cabbage, chopped

2 cups carrots, chopped

2 cups spinach, chopped

One large sweet potato, cubed

2 cups eggplant, thinly sliced

One teaspoon parsley

One teaspoon oregano

1 cup frozen peas

One teaspoon black pepper

Four large tomatoes, quartered

6 cups vegetable broth

½ teaspoon paprika

½ teaspoon

Three tablespoons extra virgin olive oil

Sea salt

Directions

- To a large pot, add the olive oil and sauté the onions, garlic, and the turkey. Cook over medium heat for 8 – 10 minutes.
- Add the kale, carrot, potatoes and frozen peas. Cook for another 2 minutes.
- Pour in the eggplant, tomatoes, spinach, and spices. Stir well before pouring in the broth.
- Cover pot and bring to a boil.
- Reduce the heat and allow simmering for 25 – 30 minutes.
- Serve warm.

Barbecued Parsley Beef Burgers

Ingredients

½ cup fresh parsley

Four tablespoon barbecue sauce

1 ½ pound lean beef

Two cloves garlic, minced

Eight whole wheat burger buns

2 cups bread crumbs

One teaspoon black pepper

One small onion, chopped

One tomato, sliced

Two tablespoons extra virgin olive oil

½ teaspoon oregano

Sea salt

Directions

- Add all the spices and bread crumbs to a large bowl and combine well. Add the beef and mix well with your hands.
- Form reasonably sized patties.
- Cook the patties on medium to high heat for 5 – 7 minutes on each side.
- Grill the buns 1 minute on cut each side.

- Put the patty on the bun and top with some cheese.

Quinoa Banana Pancakes

Ingredients

Two large bananas

Four large organic eggs

½ cup whole wheat flour

¾ cup all-purpose flour

Two tablespoons extra virgin olive oil

3 cups full cream milk

½ teaspoon nutmeg

½ teaspoon black pepper

Three teaspoons baking powder

Two tablespoons honey

½ teaspoon of cocoa powder

Sea salt

Directions

- Add the whole wheat flour, all-purpose flour, sea salt, spices and baking powder to a bowl and combine well with your hands.
- Whisk the eggs, mashed bananas, and milk. Add the cocoa powder, and then gradually introduce the flour.
- Apply some butter to a large skillet over medium heat. Pour ½ cup of batter into the skillet and cook until the bottom is brown, then turn over and cook too.
- Serve warm with honey.

Chapter Five

Spicy Chicken Tacos

Ingredients

1 pound chicken breast fillet

One teaspoon oregano

One teaspoon jalapeno

½ teaspoon rosemary

½ teaspoon ginger powder

Two cloves garlic, minced

Ten corn tortillas

2 cups chopped lettuce

Five tablespoons lime juice

One tablespoon parsley

Sea salt

Directions

- To a bowl, add the first six ingredients. Whisk thoroughly and add the chicken fillets. Coat properly.
- Allow standing for 60 – 70 minutes in a refrigerator.
- Remove the chicken fillet out of the marinade and grill over medium heat, 6 – 8 minutes per side.
- Grill the tortillas for about 1 minute.
- Place some lettuce, grilled chicken, a dash of parsley, some lime juice and fold the tortilla.
- Enjoy!

Lentil Soup

Ingredients

2 pounds lentils

Two tablespoons extra virgin olive oil

One large onion, thinly sliced

1 cup carrots, chopped

1 cup quinoa

6 cups beef broth

½ teaspoon basil

½ teaspoon rosemary

One teaspoon chili

Two tablespoons butter

1 cup broccoli, chopped

Two large tomatoes

Sea salt

Directions

- Add the olive oil, butter to a pot and sauté the vegetables over medium heat for about 5 – 7 minutes.
- Add in the quinoa, beef broth and spices. Turn the heat up, and gently bring to a boil.

- Reduce the heat and allow the mixture to simmer over low heat for 35 – 40 minutes. Stir intermittently.
- Make use of an immersion blender to blend the soup.
- Put back the pureed soup to heat for 2 - 3 minutes.
- Serve warm.

Shrimp Salad

Ingredients

1 ½ pound shrimp, uncooked

1 cup broccoli, chopped

1 cup baby spinach, chopped

Two tablespoons basil

One teaspoon cayenne pepper

Four tablespoons extra virgin olive oil

1 cup zucchini, thinly sliced

½ cup carrot, thinly sliced

One medium-sized tomato, quartered

Two cloves garlic, minced

½ teaspoon oregano

Sea salt

Directions

- Add the vegetables to a bowl, spices, and one tablespoon olive oil and toss.
- Add some spices to the shrimp and toss. Allow sitting for about 5 – 10 minutes.
- Skewer the shrimps and grill over medium heat for 3 – 5 minutes on each side.
- Remove shrimps from the skewers and serve with the salad.

Shredded Chicken Salad

Ingredients

2 pounds boneless chicken breasts

2 cups chopped green chilies

One large tomato, chopped

One large onion, chopped

Four cloves garlic, minced

One teaspoon paprika

½ cup apple cider vinegar

1 cup frozen yellow corn

1 cup mixed cheese

Two packs mixed salad greens

One can black-eyed peas

One teaspoon cayenne pepper

½ teaspoon black pepper

Salad dressing

Sea salt

Directions

- Combine peppers, spices, and vinegar in a small bowl.

- Place the chicken breasts in a slow cooker and pour the mixed spices over it.
- Cook on low heat for 5 – 7 hours.
- Remove the chicken from the slow cooker and shred using a fork.
- Combine the salad greens in a bowl and add your choice of dressing. Toss well to combine.
- Serve salad with shredded chicken topped with black-eyed peas.
- Enjoy!

Conclusion

If hypertension goes under the radar without been detected in an individual, the consequences can be quite dire. However, with the knowledge of how to modify diets can go a long way in bringing blood pressure back to normal rather than taking pills and other medications which might bring about other side effects that were not previously existing.

Bringing about a total overhaul of your lifestyle can also lower your blood pressure significantly, and such ways include going on a diet rich in vegetables, fruits, low in sodium, engaging in regular exercise, reducing alcohol intake and so much more. With our ever busy lifestyles, taking a breather, letting off steam and taking charge of your stress levels also helps.

If you have decided to take the journey towards normalizing your blood pressure, the first step is making changes to your diet and other lifestyle changes. With your mind made up, you may still find it challenging getting the foods that will do the trick. Building a relationship with the menus and recipes in this book is the solution to getting rid of the excess weight and your blood pressure problems. Food is medicinal and loving the right type of food holds so much power.

Start this healthy journey with whole, nourishing foods with your very next meal.

The Holistic Whole Food Diet Cookbook for Everyone

Healthy Tasty Recipes to Boost your Metabolism, Energize your Body and Achieve Maximum Weight Loss

By

Rina S. Gritton

Acknowledgements

This book could not have been written without the guidance and generosity of many people. To all of you who encouraged and stood by me, thank you. To my wonderful friend Lee Ryce thanks for your constant support and encouragement.

Copyright © 2019 Rina S. Gritton

The author retains all rights. No part of this document may be reproduced or transmitted in any form or by any means, electronic or mechanical, including photocopying, recording, or by any information storage and retrieval system without permission in writing from the author. The unauthorized reproduction or distribution of this copyrighted work is illegal.

Disclaimer

The information contained in this material is based on years of several types of research by scientists, dieticians and other professionals in the health field. Whatever you read within the pages of this book is for purely of informational purposes only and is not to be taken as a guide for diagnosis for any psychological or medical condition, nor to treat, mitigate or prevent any disease. Do not discard the professional advice from qualified health care personnel based on the information you get from this book. This book is not intended to be, and you should decide your health based on appropriate discussions with a qualified medical doctor or healthcare professional.

"Let medicine be your food and food thy medicine"~ Hippocrates

INTRODUCTION

We have got quite a lot of food groups all over the place that we consume without giving a second thought about, but they are having a significant deleterious effect on your wellbeing with you been unaware of the damage been done. You might have continuously suffered from severe pains, constant cold, gastrointestinal disorders, etc. and it never seems to go away even with the best treatments available. You have tried to narrow down what the cause might be, gone for several tests and nothing came up. The problem can almost certainly be from the food that you eat day in day out. So how do you go about been sure of the cause of your ailments? Begin to remove certain food items out of your daily meals.

Start by dumping all those food items with excessive amounts of calories, those food items that alter the composition and number of healthy gut bacteria, food that lack any nutritional value, etc. Going down this route will give your system a reboot and the opportunity to begin to heal.

The importance of consuming whole foods cannot be overemphasized, your general outlook on what goes into your body will change forever, your taste buds will undergo rejuvenation, what you look forward to eating at any time of the day will drastically change. All these will inevitably bring about a healthy relationship with your food and the entirety of your whole being. Incorporating and bringing whole foods to the table will bring about a positive turnaround in the way you and your loved ones come to see food for good.

Going about changing your diets and the way you relate with your food can be a daunting task which not many people will readily embark upon. A few people will stop halfway with only the hardy and determined going through with this lifestyle and reaping the benefits. For you to begin with the relationship with healthy whole food diets, you can start gradually with a 30 days program to build the foundation of the friendship you are about to have with these food types. Here are some of the simple basics that you need to help you on your journey.

Be Aware and Prepare

In this month of eating entirely whole foods and no trash, it is crucial that you continue with your daily activities and life in general. It is essential that you make no drastic changes to your schedules, social, etc. If you are to have a dinner or party with friends from the office if it's possible, try having a look at the meals that will be served at such gatherings. Having an idea of what is going to be on offer will give you time to prepare and work out a strategy of dealing with the situation. Some food items on the menu may not comply with the whole food diet, and you can make substitutions by getting alternatives before you sit at the table. Such situations are even easier to handle when you have informal social gatherings with friends. You can merely overlook some dishes and go with those you know more beneficial to your system. Your headspace will be clearer of clutter when you walk into such a place.

Your Loved Ones

It is imperative that folks around you are aware of this new dietary plan you are on because their backing and encouragement will go a long way in urging you on towards your eventual goal. As you move along with the whole food diet, your joy at been healthy and radiant outlook on life will most certainly bring about new converts too! The more, the merrier to join the bandwagon of eating whole healthy foods. So you going out on a night out with some friends who joke around a lot, it will be wise to have someone supportive to tag along with you who will give you words of encouragement and stand up for you when the taunts start to fly in. Such a person will also be a voice or reason especially when you are about to fall off the wagon. Such a person should not be too far from you, preferably your partner, sister or brother, a person that you can rely on to be there for you at all times.

Now you have made up your mind to have a healthy relationship with food; you have some of the following activities lined up for you to ease your way gently into the whole food program.

Shopping

Arrange your trips to the grocery shop every week and do not shop on impulse. Always have a checklist of all that you will need before heading out. Do not over shop at any given time to avoid wastage of the food and your funds!

Preparation

After you have gotten your stuff home, clean them and store as appropriate. This will make it easier for you to prepare when cooking and cut down on the cooking time especially during the week when you have heavy work schedules. This will make your dinner preparations a breeze and something you will not dread.

The Size

After you must have prepared some meals that you intend preserving, always use the appropriately sized containers for a single meal. You pick a bowl of food during the week, microwave it and you are good to go! Life cannot just be more comfortable!

Don'ts

To obtain the most advantage out of the whole food diets, it is important not to compromise on what you eat during this period and eventually becoming a habit. Focusing on nourishing and life-giving healthy whole foods will give you a new lease on life by reducing your digestive system issues, those bone-jarring pains that rip through your joints, the skin inflammations, etc. To be fit at all time and improve your quality of life, you should as a point of note, avoid the following "food" types. Avoid the following for this period; alcohol, processed foods, legumes, food additives like MSG, white potatoes, grains, dairy, etc.

Health Benefits

So after much consideration, you have decided to give the whole diet lifestyle a shot. It will not just help with getting rid and maintaining a healthy weight; it goes a long way in negating the debilitating effects and risks associated with specific diseases. Here are a few and not limited to the benefits linked to a whole diet plan.

Cardiac Disease

The fact that whole foods reduce the chances of coming down with a heart attack is well known. It should be known that the food choices you make concerning this is very vital. There are abundant records of individuals who have stuck to a whole food diet and are experiencing a new lease of life almost devoid of the risks of heart disease. The inclusion of highly processed foods is most likely a precursor to severe heart conditions.

Decline in Cognitive Abilities

Meals and diet types which are based on whole foods, fruits, and vegetables when consumed regularly tends to slow down the onset or cut out the chances of certain cognitive diseases. The presence of certain substances in whole foods slows down drastically the rate of cognitive defects and may even reverse damages done already.

Prevention of Gastrointestinal Disorders

Your gut microbes and flora will maintain a healthy balance which will prevent any occurrence of a gut disorder like a leaky gut. Whole foods aid the right balance of microbes and promote the formation of short-chain fatty acids that dramatically improves the blood sugar levels. Most spices and herbs are great prebiotics that will always keep your gut in top condition.

Dental Health

When you eat foods that contain less refined sugars, your teeth will not experience decay and other dental problems. The regular intake of whole foods like green tea and cheese has been shown to prevent the deterioration of the enamel significantly and to harden it. If you are a soda addict, the chances that you are already suffering from tooth decay or will come down with cavities is very high.

Diabetes

Going with a whole food diet may be the only option that you have in preventing the onset of diabetes or getting a grip on it.

Clear Skin

The whole food diet is not just right for your overall internal health. It also makes your skin glow and healthy. Cocoa-based products that have not undergone too much refining have been shown to protect against UV radiation. The elasticity and the radiance of your skin can also be improved and maintained by the consumption of olive oil, nuts, fish, etc.

The Grind

This 30 days of focusing entirely on eating whole foods to get your system in top shape without throwing in the towel halfway through is one of a kind decision that I must tell you won't be easy especially for the faint of heart. Right before you start, you should have it at the back of your mind that the whole diet lifestyle is natural! It is all about your mindset, and if you see it as a challenge, then you will have a lot of barriers to overcome which may drain you mentally and physically. When you sit down to think about it, giving up a lot of your bad habits can be downright hard because your body has become so dependent on such substances. With eating right, it involves walking away from a lot of harmful food substances, and you should not shy away from it. When you consider it, it is only for a few days, one day after the other and before you know it, the thirty days are over with your system back in tip-top shape and rearing to go!

Now you have to avoid some "empty" foods and additives. You must build up your personality and have the gut to walk away and kindly decline some offers especially when the situation becomes tempting. Get some steel in you and walk away. You certainly do not have to be afraid of hurting some feelings, e.g. your parents are having their 30th wedding anniversary, and there is a spread out in the garden with drinks and all. You have to brave up and chose your way carefully around this minefield. Do not be shamed into eating what you do not want to eat. Pick what you know is advantageous to your body and leave the rest.

There is no room for you making a mistake during this period and drinking a bottle of vodka thinking its water! Or you are heaping two full tablespoons of sugar into your coffee! You have come this far with your ultimate goal of losing some excess weight and getting your system in the best shape ever. You were not coerced into the diet plan, nor were you deceived. You made an informed decision, and it will do you a whole lot of good to stick to the program for the duration. Do not let any doubts on your staying power creep into your mind. You started it, and you can finish it!

Since this diet requires you avoiding certain food types, it might be a little hard; I must tell you that. You will have to get healthy alternatives for those kinds of stuff you are letting go. The new food items have to have healthy nutrients all in the right proportions. Eat enough for your body weight and take in the right amount of calories needed for your daily activities. You will have to make a well-detailed plan on what you eat at any time of the day. It is your body, your choice, and the decision on what you eat at any point in time.

Despite the change which you may find hard and reluctant to make, we have it in us to adapt to changes, and you can most certainly do this. You have thought about this, researched and seen the health benefits you can gain. You cannot back out now. The moment you stop considering and take an informed action will be the best decision you ever made for your body.

CHAPTER ONE

Roasted Duck

Ingredients

One whole duck

One teaspoon fresh parsley

One clove garlic, crushed

One small onion, chopped

One small bell pepper, sliced

½ teaspoon dried rosemary

½ teaspoon black pepper

Two tablespoons ghee

One tablespoon extra virgin olive oil

One lemon, sliced

One large carrot, cubed

One large sweet potato, peeled and cubed

Sea salt

Directions

- Preheat oven to 350°C.
- Combine the spices, herbs, vegetables, and seasonings in a bowl.
- Fill the duck with the vegetable mixture.
- Secure the legs of the duck together using twine.
- Soften the ghee and olive oil.
- Thoroughly bask the duck with the oil mixture.
- Place the duck in a roasting pan.
- Roast for about 75 – 90 minutes.
- Check intermittently to know when it is done.
- Serve warm.

Black-eyed Peas

Ingredients

2 cups black-eyed peas

One clove garlic, minced

One small onion, chopped

One teaspoon chili

Two tablespoons extra virgin olive oil

Sea salt

Water

Directions

- Cook the beans in boiling water with a pinch of salt for about 30 minutes until is soft.
- Add the spices, pepper and olive oil.
- Cook for another 12 - 15 minutes or until the water begins to dry.
- Stir and mash using a wooden laden.
- Serve warm with some parsley or sage sprinkled on it.

Sweet Potatoes Veggies

Three large sweet potatoes, peeled and cubed

One medium-sized eggplant

2 cups vegetable broth

¼ teaspoon thyme

¼ teaspoon cilantro

½ teaspoon jalapeno

1 cup carrots, chopped

Two tablespoons extra virgin olive oil

Sea salt

Directions

- Boil the potatoes in some water until it is thoroughly soft.
- Put the potatoes into a large bowl and add the other ingredients to it.
- Using a wooden spoon, stir and combine thoroughly until a smooth, creamy mixture is obtained.
- Serve topped with some healthy salad.

Tuna Poached Eggs

Ingredients

Four large tuna fillets, cleaned and skinless

Four large organic eggs

½ teaspoon basil

½ teaspoon black pepper

½ teaspoon sage

1 cup hollandaise sauce

Four tablespoons extra virgin olive oil

Directions

- Preheat oven to 240°C.
- Spice the tuna fillets well.
- Add some oil to a large saucepan over medium heat.
- Add the fillets to the saucepan and allow cooking in the oil for 4 to 5 minutes then flipping over and allowing the other side to cook for the same period too.
- Move the baking pan into the oven and bake for about 5 minutes.

- Poach the egg in a separate pan and then move the tuna and eggs to a plate.
- Top the tuna and eggs with some hollandaise.
- Sprinkle the herbs and spices over it and enjoy!

Hollandaise

2 cups clarified salted ghee

Three tablespoons fresh lemon juice

¼ teaspoon jalapeno

Six large organic eggs

Directions

- Melt your ghee over low to medium heat in a large saucepan.
- Add the spices, egg yolks and other ingredients to a high powered blender.
- Blitz for about 30 seconds.
- Add the ghee slowly to the egg mixture while blending at reduced speed.

- Add some warm water if the consistency of the mixture becomes too thick.
- Serve warm right away!

Rabbit Cacciatore

Ingredients

2-pound rabbit thighs

Six tablespoons extra virgin olive oil

2 cups vegetable broth

One teaspoon black pepper

One large onion, thinly sliced

1 cup carrot, cubed

1 cup green peas

Two cloves garlic, crushed

One large yellow bell pepper, sliced

Two large tomatoes, diced

One tablespoon, parsley

One tablespoon cilantro

Sea salt

Directions

- In a saucepan over medium heat with three tablespoons of extra virgin olive oil, brown the spiced rabbit for 5 minutes on each side. Remove from the heat and keep.
- Add some olive oil to the pan and sauté the vegetables, spices, and herbs for about 2 minutes.
- Add the rabbits back to the saucepan with the vegetables, pour in the broth and cover.
- Allow simmering for about 35 – 45 minutes.
- Serve warm with your choice of dish.

CHAPTER TWO
Chipotle Coconut Chicken Burgers

Ingredients

½ cup coconut, grated

1 pound ground chicken meat

½ cup artichoke, chopped

One teaspoon allspice

One small onion, thinly sliced

One clove garlic, crushed

Two tablespoons extra virgin olive oil

Sea salt

Directions

- Preheat oven to 270°C.
- Mix all the ingredients but not the olive oil in a bowl using your hands.
- Forms reasonably sized balls and flatten into shape using your hands.

- Apply some olive oil to a large saucepan.
- Place the patties in the olive oil and heat each side for about 2 minutes.
- Place the patties on a baking pan and bake for about 10 – 12 minutes.
- Serve with whole wheat bread.

Parsley Basil Pistachio Pesto

Ingredients

1 cup parsley, chopped

2 cups spinach, chopped

1 cup walnuts, roasted

1 cup basil chopped

Three tablespoons lemon juice

2 cups extra virgin olive oil

Two cloves garlic, minced

1 ½ cup shelled pistachios

½ teaspoon chipotle

Sea salt

Directions

- Add all the elements to a food processor.
- Pulse until all ingredients are chopped.
- Gradually add the olive oil and blitz until it is smooth and creamy.
- Pour into a bowl and mix in the lemon juice.
- Enjoy!

Veal Arugula Veggies

Ingredients

One medium-sized honeydew, cubed

Two bunch fresh arugula

Six pieces of veal

Two tablespoons walnuts, roasted and crushed

½ teaspoon black pepper

½ teaspoon fresh cilantro

Two tablespoons extra virgin olive oil

Sea salt

Directions

- Over medium heat in a pan, prepare the veal in olive oil for 5 minutes on each side. Take off the heat and allow cooling.
- Cut the veal into cube sizes.
- Toss the veal, honeydew, and other ingredients into a bowl.
- Combine well.
- Serve with your favorite dish and enjoy!

Pork Patties with Veggies and Mashed Sweet Potatoes

Ingredients

2 pounds ground pork

½ teaspoon chipotle

½ teaspoon dried basil

One small onion, thinly sliced

One clove garlic, minced

½ teaspoon curry

One teaspoon thyme

½ teaspoon coriander

Three large sweet potatoes, cubed

Six tablespoons clarified butter

1 cup full cream milk

1 cup green peas, frozen

1 cup carrots, cubed

1 cup eggplant, thinly sliced

2 cups spinach, chopped

1 cup kale, chopped

One teaspoon black pepper

Sea salt

Two tablespoons extra virgin olive oil

Two tablespoons, lemon zest

Directions

- Preheat oven to 245°C.
- Pour the pork into a large bowl and add all the spices, salt, and herbs.
- Combine well using your hands.
- Form patties and store in a freezer for 15 – 20 minutes.
- Add the sweet potatoes to a pot of water and boil until very tender.
- Strain out the water leaving the potatoes.
- Add the full cream milk and butter.
- Mash well until smooth and creamy.
- Seal the pot and keep.
- Arrange the pork on a foil-lined baking pan.
- Bake for 15 – 20 minutes.
- Add olive oil to a pan over medium heat, sauté the onions, garlic, and the veggies. Stir well for about 2 – 4 minutes.
- Add the sautéed vegetables to the mashed

potatoes and stir.
- Serve the mashed potatoes with the baked pork patties warm.
- Enjoy!

Grilled BBQ Turkey Wings

Ingredients

12 large turkey wings

Homemade BBQ sauce

Ingredients

Four cloves garlic, crushed

One teaspoon chipotle

One large onion, blended

1 cup tomato paste

½ teaspoon black pepper

½ teaspoon cilantro

½ teaspoon paprika

½ teaspoon oregano

½ cup mustard

One tablespoon apple cider vinegar

Six tablespoons extra virgin olive oil

Six dates pitted

Six large tomatoes, blended

Directions

BBQ Sauce

- Add all the individual ingredients to a large pot.
- Cook on low heat for about 10 – 15 minutes.
- Stir intermittently.
- Introduce all the contents of the pot into a food processor.
- Pulse until everything is smooth.
- Pour the contents into a mason jar and refrigerate or make use of it immediately.

Homemade BBQ marinade

Ingredients

2 ½ tablespoons garlic powder

One teaspoon oregano

½ tablespoon paprika

One tablespoon dried cilantro

One tablespoon dried basil

One tablespoon fresh parsley

½ teaspoon jalapeno

½ teaspoon black pepper

One teaspoon chili

Sea salt

Directions

- Pour the ingredients into a container and combine well.
- Pour into a jar and seal.

- Shake well and keep on your kitchen cabinet.

Grilled Turkey Wings

Directions

- Preheat oven to 275°C.
- Line the baking pans with baking foils.
- Thoroughly dowse and toss each wing in the marinade and sauce.
- Bake for 25 – 30 minutes.
- Serve warm with a side of salad.

CHAPTER THREE
Grilled Chicken with Chipotle-Kale puree and Green peas

Ingredients

Eight chicken breasts

One teaspoon chili

Three cloves garlic, minced

2 cups green peas

2 cups kale, chopped

One teaspoon chipotle

1 cup carrot, cubed

1 cup zucchini, sliced

Four tablespoons extra virgin olive oil

½ teaspoon paprika

½ teaspoon cilantro

Sea salt

Directions

- Preheat the grill to 395°C and oven to 270°C.
- Combine some chili, garlic, and salt. Use the mixture to cover the chicken breasts.
- Combine the vegetables, spices, herbs and olive oil in a bowl. Arrange on a baking foil and bake for 30 minutes.
- Pour the roasted vegetables into a blender, add some olive oil and blitz.
- Add the green peas to the blended mixture and mix.
- Grill the chicken to your taste.
- Put the grilled chicken breasts on a plate and pour the blended vegetables over the chicken breasts and enjoy!

Spicy Crab Meat and Eggplant Noodles

Ingredients

2 pounds crab meat, cooked

Six cups eggplant "noodles."

Four tablespoons extra virgin olive oil

Three cloves garlic, minced

One large onion, sliced

One teaspoon jalapeno

One teaspoon fresh cilantro, chopped

One teaspoon fresh basil, chopped

½ teaspoon soy sauce

Sea salt

Directions

- Peel the eggplant, and then make use of a spiral slicer. Keep the noodles.
- Sauté the onions and garlic in olive oil over medium heat for about two minutes.
- Add the crab meats, spices and herbs to the sautéed onions and stir well.
- Add some water to the crab meat. Allow simmering for about 10 minutes.
- Pour into a bowl.

- Steam the eggplant noodles using a colander for about 2 minutes.
- Serve the noodles in a flat plate and top with some crab meat.
- Enjoy!

Arugula Salad

Ingredients

6 cups arugula, chopped

Two tablespoons vinegar

Two tablespoons flax seeds

1 ½ cup mayonnaise

¼ cup blueberries

One small tomato, sliced

One small onion, sliced

1 cup kale, sliced

½ teaspoon basil

½ teaspoon cilantro

Sea salt

Directions

- Add all the ingredients to a large container.
- Toss and stir well with a wooden spoon until the vegetables are thoroughly coated with the mayonnaise.
- Add the vinegar and stir.
- Add some salt to taste.
- Serve and enjoy.

Grilled Veggies and Fruits

Ingredients

Two large apples, cored and sliced

Four tablespoons extra virgin olive oil

2 cups mixed berries

1 cup banana, sliced

½ cup dates

1 cup carrots, cubed

1 cup zucchini, sliced

½ teaspoon chipotle

½ teaspoon allspice

1 cup almond, crushed and roasted

Sea salt

Directions

- Add the olive oil and spices to a bowl and combine well. Set aside.
- Add the fruits and vegetables to the olive oil mixture.
- Combine well.
- Grill the fruits for about 2 -3 minutes.
- Serve warm sprinkled with almond.

Fried Salmon

Ingredients

Four salmon fillets

Three tablespoons extra virgin olive oil

½ teaspoon oregano

½ teaspoon paprika

½ teaspoon black pepper

Sea salt

Directions

- Combine the spices in a bowl and thoroughly cover the salmon fillets with the spices.
- Allow the fillet marinade in the spices for about an hour.
- Add some olive oil to a skillet over medium heat.
- Introduce the salmon to the olive oil and allow each side to cook until it turns a shade of light pink.
- Serve with your choice of salad.
- Enjoy!

Spicy Deviled Eggs

Ingredients

Eight hard-boiled organic eggs

¼ teaspoon chili

½ teaspoon garlic powder

½ teaspoon onion powder

One tablespoon extra virgin olive oil

¼ teaspoon paprika

Three tablespoons mayonnaise

One teaspoon basil, chopped

Sea salt

Directions

- Peel the boiled eggs and slice them halfway longitudinally.
- Remove the yolks and keep in a small bowl.
- To the yolks, add all the spices.
- Combine thoroughly using a fork.
- Scoop back the yolks into the egg white.
- Sprinkle some basil over the deviled eggs.

Sautéed Vegetables

Ingredients

2 cups spinach, chopped

2 cups kale, chopped

1 cup carrot, chopped

1 cup zucchini, thinly sliced

One clove garlic, minced

One large onion, thinly sliced

One teaspoon chili

One teaspoon rosemary

½ teaspoon sage

½ teaspoon oregano

1 cup green peas

Two tablespoons extra virgin olive oil

Sea salt

Directions

- Add some oil to a large pan.
- Sauté the onions and garlic for about minutes until translucent.
- Add the vegetables and continue to stir for about 1 minute.
- Add the herbs and spices and cook for another minute.
- Serve warm.

CHAPTER FOUR
SOUPS

Roasted Brussels Sprout and Carrot Soup

Ingredients

3 cups Brussels sprouts, cleaned

2 cups carrots, chopped

One large onion, thinly sliced

Four tablespoons extra virgin olive oil

1 cup yellow corn, cooked

Four cloves garlic, minced

3 cups chicken broth

One teaspoon chili

One red bell pepper, thinly sliced

½ teaspoon turmeric

½ teaspoon sage

½ teaspoon coriander

1 cup black-eyed peas, cooked

One teaspoon cilantro

One teaspoon basil

Sea salt

Directions

- Preheat oven to 265°C.
- Add some olive oil, turmeric, chili, bell pepper, and spices to a bowl.
- Combine well and add the carrots, sprouts, and corn.
- Toss well to coat the vegetables.
- Arrange the vegetables on a baking sheet.
- Roast in the oven for about 16 – 20 minutes.
- Add some olive oil to a saucepan over medium heat.
- Sauté the garlic and onions for about 1 minute. Stir continuously.

- Pour in the broth to a food processor; add the sautéed onions and vegetables.
- Pulse and blitz until your desired consistency are achieved.
- Sprinkle some basil and cilantro on it and enjoy!

Sweet Potato Ginger Soup

Two large sweet potatoes, cleaned and cubed

One tablespoon ginger, grated

One teaspoon turmeric

One teaspoon curry

½ teaspoon thyme

6 cups vegetable broth

Three tablespoons extra virgin olive oil

2 cups lentils

½ teaspoon oregano

½ teaspoon jalapeno

1 cup full cream milk

Sea salt

Directions

- Preheat oven to 295°C.
- Combine the vegetables, spices and herbs, olive oil in a bowl.
- Pour the content of the bowl onto a baking pan lined with baking sheet.
- Bake for 15 – 20 minutes and stir intermittently.
- Pour the roasted vegetables to a large pot and add the broth.
- Boil at high heat, and then allow simmering for 8 – 10 minutes.
- Introduce the contents of the pot into a food processor.
- Blend until smooth and then add the full cream milk.
- Serve warm or allow cooling in the fridge before serving.

Turmeric Lentil Soup

Ingredients

3 cups lentils

One teaspoon turmeric

One shallot, chopped

5 cups vegetable broth

¼ teaspoon nutmeg

One teaspoon basil

1 cup arugula, chopped

One tablespoon curry powder

Two cloves garlic, minced

1 ½ cup full cream milk

Three tablespoons extra virgin olive oil

Sea salt

Directions

- In a large skillet, sauté the vegetables for 2 minutes in olive oil over medium heat.
- Add the spices and broth.
- Allow simmering for about 20 minutes.
- Add the milk and simmer for another 3 minutes.
- Serve warm.

Eggplant Cilantro Soup

3 pounds eggplant, thinly sliced

5 cups chicken broth

1 ½ cup white wine

½ cup extra virgin olive oil

½ cup cilantro, packed

½ teaspoon black pepper

One large onion, thinly sliced

2 cloves garlic, crushed

½ teaspoon rosemary

Sea salt

Directions

- Sauté garlic and onions in olive oil over medium heat for 3 – 5 minutes. Stir.
- Add eggplant and continue to stir.
- Pour in the wine and broth.
- Allow simmering for 10 – 15 minutes.
- Add cilantro and take the pot off the heat.
- Add spices and herbs.
- Add the vegetable to a food processor and blend.
- Serve warm.

Spinach and Brown Bean Soup

Ingredients

200g boneless chicken breast, cubed

Three cloves garlic, minced

Two tablespoons extra virgin olive oil

2 cups vegetable broth

2 cups spinach, packed

2 cups brown beans, cooked

One large onion, thinly sliced

One red bell pepper, sliced

One teaspoon cilantro

One teaspoon basil

½ teaspoon paprika

Two large tomatoes, chopped

Sea salt

Directions

- Add the olive oil to a pot over medium heat.
- Add the chicken breasts and cook for 5 – 10 minutes. Stir continuously.
- Add the onions and garlic, sauté for another 3 – 5 minutes.
- Introduce the beans, spinach, spices, and herbs. Stir and pour in the broth.

- Cook for 2 minutes.
- Use an immersion blender to blitz until creamy.
- Serve warm.

Lentil Soup

4 cups lentil

1 cup carrots, cubed

1 cup kale, chopped

Two cloves garlic

5 cups low sodium chicken broth

Three tablespoons extra virgin olive oil

Two tablespoons flax seeds

½ tablespoon apple cider vinegar

½ teaspoon chili

 Sea salt

Directions

- Add the vegetables to a pot and pour in the broth.
- Heat on high heat till it boils then reduce heat to allow simmering for 5 minutes.
- Add the spices, herbs and other ingredients.
- Pour into a blender when it is cool and blend until smooth.
- Serve with some garlic bread or toppings of your choice.

CHAPTER FIVE
SEAFOOD, MEAT AND POULTRY

Chipotle-spiced Veal with Veggies

Ingredients

One tablespoon extra virgin olive oil

1 pound veal roast

1 cup carrots, chopped

1 cup kale, chopped

1 cup onions, diced

2 cups spinach, packed

One large zucchini, thinly sliced

1 cup green peas

Two cloves garlic, minced

½ cup fresh cilantro, chopped

½ cup fresh basil, chopped

½ teaspoon ginger, grated

One teaspoon thyme

1 ½ tablespoon lemon juice, fresh

½ teaspoon allspice

1 ½ teaspoon cinnamon

½ teaspoon paprika

One tablespoon chipotle

½ teaspoon coriander

½ teaspoon red wine vinegar

½ teaspoon black pepper

Sea salt

Directions

- Preheat oven to 285°C.
- Add all the chopped vegetables to a bowl; add some lemon juice, salt, and vinegar.
- Toss well to combine correctly.
- Keep in the fridge.
- Add the veal, spices, and herbs to a bowl.

Use your hand to distribute the seasoning evenly.
- Allow marinating for about 60 minutes.
- Place the veal on a baking foil in a baking pan.
- Bake for 15 – 20 minutes or until done to your taste.
- Allow cooling,
- Serve with the vegetables.

Stir-fried Duck

1 ½ pound duck breast, cubed, boneless and skinless

1 ½ bag frozen mixed vegetable stir-fry

Two tablespoons extra virgin olive oil

Two cloves garlic, minced

One large onion, thinly sliced

½ tablespoon oregano

½ tablespoon soy sauce

½ teaspoon basil

½ teaspoon black pepper

Three tablespoons cornstarch

Two egg white, beaten

½ cup vegetable broth

Sea salt

Directions

- Sauté garlic and onions in olive oil over medium heat in a large saucepan for about 1 minute.
- Place the egg white in one bowl and the cornstarch in a separate bowl.
- Dip the cubed duck breast into the egg white and then the cornstarch.
- Put the duck into the oiled pan and stir fry for 7 – 10 minutes.
- Add the spices, soy sauce, oregano, broth, etc.
- Allow to boil, and then let it simmer.

- Introduce the vegetables and stir.
- Allow cooking on low heat for 4 – 5 minutes.
- Serve warm in bowls.

Barca Kabobs

Ingredients

Kabobs

1 pound lean beef, cubed

1 pound turkey breast, boneless and skinless, cubed

One large red onion, cubed

One large green bell pepper, chopped

Six large tomatoes, quartered

Wooden skewers, soaked in water for some minutes

Marinade

Three tablespoons extra virgin olive oil

Two cloves garlic, minced

One tablespoon basil, fresh

One tablespoon cilantro, fresh

½ teaspoon chili

Sea salt

Directions

- Preheat oven to 290°C.
- Add all the individual ingredients for the marinade in a bowl. Combine well then halve it into two separate bowls.
- To one bowl of the marinade, add the turkey, beef, tomatoes, onion, green pepper.
- Wash away the used marinade.
- Let it marinade for 15 – 20 minutes.
- Skewer the beef, turkey, onions, pepper, tomatoes alternatively on a wooden skewer.
- Grill for 10 – 15 minutes while turning the

skewers continuously.
- Serve warm and apply some of the other half of the marinade on the kabobs.

Nagasaki Beef Noodle Soup

Ingredients

Meat and Veggies

Two bags frozen mixed vegetable stir-fry

2 pounds lean beef, thinly sliced

One pack noodles

2 cups scallions, diced

1 cup kale, chopped

One red onion, thinly sliced

One clove garlic, minced

1 cup tofu

Broth

6 cups low sodium beef broth

1 ½ tablespoon soy sauce

Two cloves garlic, minced

One tablespoon ginger, minced

2 cups mushrooms stems, washed and cleaned

One tablespoon lemon zest, fresh

½ teaspoon parsley

Directions

- To a saucepan, add all the ingredients for the broth except for the soy sauce. Allow boiling then reduce the heat to low heat and let it simmer for 10 – 15 minutes.
- Drain the liquid part of the broth into a container and throw away the solids.
- Return the broth to heat; add the soy sauce, mushrooms, and vegetables.
- Let simmer on low heat for about 2 minutes.
- Introduce the noodles and let it cook on

low heat for another 1 – 2 minutes.
- Put in the beef.
- Cook for 5 – 10 minutes.
- Add kale, tofu, and scallions.
- Cook for a further 2 minutes.
- Serve warm.
- Enjoy!

Spicy Pork Casserole

Ingredients

1 pound ground pork

One large red bell pepper, sliced

2 cups green peas

One large carrot, diced

Two large tomatoes, diced

One large white onion, thinly sliced

½ teaspoon black pepper

½ teaspoon cinnamon

½ teaspoon paprika

1 ½ cup brown rice, uncooked

2 cups of water

One tablespoon extra virgin olive oil

Sea salt

Directions

- Add the pork to a saucepan over medium heat and sauté it until slightly brown.
- Strain the fat from the pork.
- Introduce the other ingredients into the pan and sauté.
- Let it cook over medium heat until it begins to boil.
- Turn down the heat.
- Let simmer for 45 – 50 minutes.
- Serve hot and enjoy!

Beef sirloin with spicy tomato sauce

Ingredients

1 pound lean beef

Two tablespoons extra virgin olive oil

Three cloves garlic, minced

2 cups tomatoes, diced

2 cups scallions, diced

One tablespoon tomato paste

1 cup mushroom, washed and cleaned

3 cups vegetable broth

One tablespoon red wine vinegar

One large onion, thinly sliced

One tablespoon cilantro, fresh

One teaspoon parsley, dried

½ teaspoon chili

One tablespoon cornstarch

Sea salt

Directions

- Preheat oven to 290°C.
- Add some olive oil to the large saucepan over medium heat.
- Introduce to beef and gently cook both sides until brown for at least 3 – 4 minutes.
- Move the beef onto a baking sheet in a baking pan.
- Put it in the oven and let it cook for another 5 – 7 minutes.
- To the saucepan, add the onions and garlic, sauté for 1 minute.
- Put in the scallions and mushrooms and sauté for about 3 minutes over low heat.
- Add the vinegar, chopped tomatoes and tomato paste, spices, and herbs — Cook for a further 2 minutes.
- Combine the cornstarch and broth in a bowl and pour the mixture into the saucepan.
- Increase the heat and stir continuously.

- Allow simmering for 1-2 minutes.
- Serve warm with the sirloin.

Viet Chicken Curry

Ingredients

1 pound chicken breast, boneless, skinless and cut into 1" strips

1 pound mixed vegetables

Two tablespoons extra virgin olive oil

Two cloves garlic, minced

One teaspoon ginger, minced

1 cup green onions, chopped

1 cup low fat coconut milk

1 ½ tablespoon green curry paste

One tablespoon lemon zest

1 ½ teaspoon fish sauce

1 ½ teaspoon honey

1 cup chicken broth

1 ½ teaspoon soy sauce

1 ½ tablespoon cornstarch

Directions

- Heat some olive oil in a large saucepan over medium heat.
- Sauté the onions, garlic, lemon zest, and ginger for about 2 minutes.
- Put in the curry and continue to stir for 2 minutes.
- Introduce the fish sauce, coconut milk, soy sauce, and honey. Stir and cook on high heat until it begins to boil.
- Combine cornstarch and broth in a bowl and pour into the saucepan. Continue to stir on low heat.
- Put in the chicken and cook for 8 – 10 minutes.
- Pour in the mixed vegetables, stir, cover the pan and cook for about 3 minutes.

- Serve warm in bowls.

Chicken and Arugula Stir-fry

Ingredients

1 pound boneless, chicken breast, chopped into 1" strips

2 cups arugula, chopped

Two tablespoons extra virgin olive oil

Three cloves garlic, minced

One tablespoon ginger, grated

One large carrot, cut into thin pieces

1 ½ tablespoon soy sauce

One tablespoon cornstarch

2 cups vegetable broth

One large green onion, thinly sliced

One tablespoon white wine vinegar

Directions

- Stir fry onions, ginger and garlic in olive oil over medium heat for about 1 minute.
- Add arugula and carrots. Cook for 2 – 3 minutes
- Combine broth and cornstarch and pour into the pan.
- Pour in the vinegar and increase the heat until it begins to boil. Then allow simmering.
- Put in the chicken, cook for 10 minutes.

Add the soy sauce and cook for 1 minute.

- Serve warm with whole wheat pasta or some wild rice.

Oven-Crusted Turkey Breast

Ingredients

Six boneless, skinless turkey breasts, pounded into 1" thickness

1 ½ cup low-fat milk

Two egg white, lightly beaten

One tablespoon lemon juice

Three tablespoons extra virgin olive oil

1 ½ cup bread crumbs

1 ½ cup whole-wheat flour

Four large tomatoes halved

1 cup scallions, minced

One clove garlic, minced

1 cup eggplant, thinly sliced

1 cup kale, chopped

Three tablespoons oats, crushed

½ teaspoon black pepper

Sea salt

Directions

- Preheat oven to 290°C.
- Add the oats and breadcrumbs to a bowl and mix well. To another bowl, combine

the milk and egg and set aside.
- Coat the turkey breasts in whole wheat flour and remove any excess. Put the turkey in the milk mixture followed by the oat mixture.
- Heat some olive oil over medium heat in a large saucepan. Stir fry the turkey for about 3 – 5 minutes on all sides until brown.
- Remove from the heat to drain off excess oil.
- Place on baking sheets in a pan and put into the oven.
- Cook for 6 – 9 minutes.
- Combine the olive oil and lemon juice; add the tomatoes, kale, and eggplants. Toss to combine well. Sprinkle some pepper and salt.
- Serve the turkey warm and salad.
- Enjoy!

Hanoi Chicken Wraps

Ingredients

1 pound boneless chicken breast, chopped into 1" strips

Three bok choy, shredded

One tablespoon soy sauce

Four tablespoon honey

One tablespoon ginger, minced

One jalapeno pepper, deseeded and minced

One medium sized lettuce

One teaspoon fish sauce

Two tablespoons lime juice

Two cloves garlic, minced

12 fresh basil leaves

½ cup of water

Directions

- Stir fry garlic and onions in olive oil for

about 1 minute.
- Put in the chicken and stir for another 8 – 10 minutes.
- Add the soy sauce and fry for 30 seconds.
- Add all the ingredients for the sauce to a wok over high heat. Allow boiling then taking off the heat and allow sitting for about 5 minutes.
- Keep in a fridge for about 20 minutes.
- To make the wrap, lay a lettuce leave on a large plate, add some Bok choy, chicken fry, basil leaf and then seal.
- Serve the chicken wrap with some sauce.

Goat meat Mole

Ingredients

1 pound boneless goat meat

One tablespoon black pepper

1 ½ tablespoon cocoa powder

2 cups beef broth

Four cloves garlic, minced

One teaspoon allspice

One teaspoon oregano

½ teaspoon basil

½ teaspoon paprika

Three tablespoons canola oil

One tablespoon jalapeno

One large onion, chopped

Four large tomatoes, diced

Sea salt

Directions

- Preheat oven to 290°C.
- Coat the goat meat with pepper, salt, and canola oil.
- Arrange in a baking pan and cook for 20 – 25 minutes or until done.
- Add jalapeno, onions, garlic, and other

spices to a saucepan and sauté for 1 -2 minute on low heat.
- Add some canola oil and cook for 2 minutes.
- Pour in the broth, cocoa powder, and tomatoes. Allow boiling then simmer for 6 – 8 minutes.
- Remove from the heat and allow to cool.
- Pour into a food blender, blend until smooth.
- Return the pureed content of the blender to the pot and heat over low heat.
- Serve goat meat with warm mole.

Grilled Salmon with Lentils and Kale Salad

Ingredients

1 ½ pound salmon, cut into six portions

Two tablespoons extra virgin olive oil

½ teaspoon paprika

2 cups lentils

One teaspoon oregano

1 cup kale

Two tablespoons lemon juice

Two cloves garlic, minced

One large onion, chopped

Two large tomatoes, quartered

One teaspoon black pepper

½ teaspoon basil

Sea salt

Directions

- Preheat oven to 195°C.
- Add lentils, kale, black pepper, tomato, lemon juice to a bowl and toss well.
- Keep refrigerated
- Combine oregano, paprika, salt, garlic, onion, and lemon juice.

- Generously brush the salmon with the marinade.
- Allow sitting for about 20 minutes.
- Grill the salmon for about 2 – 4 minutes on each side.
- Serve the salmon warm with the salad.

Tuna Tacos

Ingredients

1 pound tuna

6 8" whole wheat tortillas

½ cup spinach

½ cup cabbage1/2 tablespoon honey

One tablespoon jalapeno pepper

½ teaspoon chili

One large onion, thinly sliced

Two cloves garlic

One tablespoon honey

One tablespoon lime juice

½ teaspoon coriander

One tablespoon cilantro

½ teaspoon basil

One tablespoon extra virgin olive oil

Sea salt

Directions

- Preheat oven to 195°C.
- Add the lime juice, chili, olive oil, coriander, and salt in a bowl and let it sit in a cold corner.
- To another bowl, add the spinach, cabbage, lime juice, honey, onion, garlic, and jalapeno pepper.
- Combine well and let the filing stand for 15 – 20 minutes.
- Arrange the tuna fillets in a large dish and pour the marinade over it.
- Arrange the tuna on a grill and cook for 3

- 5 minutes on each side or until thoroughly done.
- Arrange the tortilla on a clean flat surface and fill with tuna and salad filling.

Orleans Shrimp Stew

Ingredients

1 pound shrimp, deveined and peeled

Two tablespoons extra virgin olive oil

Two teaspoon oregano

Two large tomatoes, diced

One teaspoon paprika

1 ½ cup chicken broth

Three cloves garlic, minced

One large onion, thinly sliced

1 cup Brussels sprouts

One tablespoon basil

½ teaspoon black pepper

1 pound sweet potatoes, peeled and cubed

One teaspoon coriander

½ teaspoon jalapeno

Sea salt

Directions

- Add some olive oil to a large saucepan and sauté the onions, garlic and Brussels sprout on medium heat for about 7 – 8 minutes.
- Pour in the broth, potatoes, and tomatoes. Turn up the heat and allow the mixture to boil for about 7 – 10 minutes.
- Add the shrimp, spices, and herbs. Reduce the heat and stir.
- Cook for 5 – 7 minutes.
- Serve warm and enjoy!

Baked Bass with Spicy Sauce

Ingredients

1 pound bass fillets

Two tablespoons extra virgin olive oil

½ teaspoon black pepper

One green bell pepper, cut into finger sized sticks

One teaspoon oregano

One teaspoon basil

½ teaspoon paprika

1 cup spicy tomato paste

Two large tomatoes, diced

One clove garlic

1 cup scallions, chopped

Sea salt

Directions

- Preheat oven to 295°C.

- Heat olive oil in a large skillet.
- Add the bell pepper, scallions, and garlic.
- Sauté for about 2 minutes.
- Add the diced tomato and tomato sauce and increase the heat until it begins to boil.
- Let it simmer for about 10 – 15 minutes.
- Add the spices and herbs and allow it to cook on low heat for another 1 – 2 minutes.
- Take off the cooker and allow it to sit.
- Season each bass fillet with salt, pepper and olive oil.
- Arrange the fillet on a baking sheet and bake for 20 – 30 minutes.
- Serve the fish with a generous about of sauce.
- Enjoy!

Rainbow Trout Provencal

1 pound trout fillets

Three tablespoons extra virgin olive oil

1 cup vegetable broth

Two large tomatoes, diced

Four cloves garlic, minced

One teaspoon cilantro

One teaspoon basil

½ teaspoon chipotle

One small onion, thinly sliced

½ cup olives, sliced

Sea salt

Directions

- Sauté the trout fillets over high heat in olive oil for about 5 minutes on each side or until the fish is done.
- Remove the fish from the oil and keep.
- Pour the onions and garlic into the pan, sauté for about 60 seconds.
- Pour in the vegetable broth and increase the heat to allow boiling.

- Introduce the other ingredients then allow simmering for a few more minutes.
- Serve warm with the fish.

Bangkok Steamed Cod

Ingredients

1 pound cod fillet

½ cup scallions

1 ½ cup vegetable broth

Two cloves garlic, minced

One teaspoon soy sauce

One teaspoon ginger powder

One tablespoon extra virgin olive oil

1 cup shiitake mushrooms, washed and cleaned

Directions

- Add all the ingredients but not the fish to a large skillet.

- Boil on high heat then allow simmering for about 1 -2 minutes.
- Introduce the cod and seal the skillet.
- Allow cooking for 4 – 6 minutes.
- Serve warm.

Baked Tilapia Dijon

Ingredients

2 pounds tilapia fillet

½ cup scallions, chopped

1 ½ tablespoon lemon juice

One teaspoon dill

One teaspoon jalapeno

Two cloves garlic, minced

Three tablespoons Dijon mustard

1 ½ cup low-fat sour cream

Sea salt

Directions

- Preheat oven to 310°C.
- Lay the tilapia fillet on a baking sheet coated with cooking spray.
- Add the mustard, scallions, garlic, cream, dill and lemon juice to a bowl and combine thoroughly.
- Add a mixture of salt and pepper on the fish followed by the prepared sauce.
- Bake fish for 18 – 22 minutes.
- Serve hot!

Pork Chops in Spicy Garlic Sauce

Six bone-in pork chops

Three tablespoons extra virgin olive oil

1 ½ cup red wine

½ teaspoon chili

Four cloves garlic, minced

1 cup prunes, dried

One large onion thinly cut

½ teaspoon tarragon

Two large tomatoes, diced

Sea salt

Directions

- Brown pork chops in olive oil over medium heat for about 3 minutes on each side.
- Remove the pork from the heat.
- Add olive oil to the pan, sauté the garlic and onions for about 3 minutes.
- Add the wine and stir for about 1 – 2 minutes.
- Pour in the prunes followed by the tarragon. Stir continuously for about 60 seconds.
- Introduce back the chops to the pan. Stir and cook on low heat for 10 – 12 minutes.
- Serve hot!

Baked Chipotle Pork Chops

Ingredients

Eight center-cut pork chops

½ cup roll oats

½ cup bread crumbs

Two egg whites

One teaspoon oregano

Two teaspoon paprika

One teaspoon onion powder

Two cloves garlic, minced

1 ½ cup low fat evaporated milk

One teaspoon dry mustard

Sea salt

Directions

- Preheat oven to 290°C.
- Pour the egg white and milk into a bowl and whisk very well.

- Place the pork chops into the milk mixture for 10 – 15 minutes. Turn the other side up after about 6 – 8 minutes.
- In another bowl, combine breadcrumbs, spices, rolled oats, spices, herbs, and salt.
- Lay a baking sheet in a baking pan and coat with cooking spray.
- Take out the pork from the egg mixture and coat with the breadcrumb mixture.
- Place the pork on the baking foil and bake for 20 – 25 minutes. Flip over the pork and cook for another 10 – 15 minutes.
- Serve hot with salad.

Grilled Pork with Spicy Sauce

Ingredients

3 pounds pork tenderloin

1 ½ tablespoon soy sauce

Two cloves garlic, crushed

1 ½ tablespoon fish sauce

½ teaspoon oregano

One teaspoon paprika

One teaspoon brown sugar

One teaspoon cayenne

Sea salt

Directions

- Preheat oven to 290°C.
- Combine all the spices, herbs and salt in a bowl.
- Clean the pork and cut out any fat.
- Apply the sauce generously over the pork.
- Let it marinade for 15 – 20 minutes.
- Grill in the oven while occasionally brushing with some marinade.
- Cook the pork for 30 – 40 minutes.
- Carve and serve the pork hot.

CHAPTER SIX
JUICES

Zesty Carrot Juice

Ingredients

Four large carrots, cubed

Two tablespoons lemon zest

2 ½ cups water

Ice cubes

Directions

- Place all the ingredients in a blender.
- Blitz at high speed until smooth.
- Serve chilled.

Tropic Delight

Ingredients

Two large bananas

One large carrot

½ cup prune

½ cup figs

1 cup mixed berries

½ teaspoon cardamom

Two tablespoons honey

½ pineapple, cubed

1 cup of water

Ice cubes

Directions

- Put all the ingredients into a blender.
- Blend at high speed until it is creamy smooth.
- Serve chilled.

Banana Berry Juice

Ingredients

Two large ripe bananas

1 cup mixed berries

One tablespoon honey

1 cup full cream strawberry yogurt

1 cup of water

Ice cubes

Directions

- Add all the ingredients to the blender.
- Secure the top.
- Blend at high speed until smooth.
- Serve chilled.

Orange Apple Juice

Ingredients

Two oranges, peeled

One large apple, cored and sliced

½ cup blackberry

½ cup of water

Ice cubes

Directions

- Put all the ingredients into the blender.
- Blend at high speed.
- Serve chilled.

Green Carrot Juice

Ingredients

One large carrot, cubed

½ cup kale

½ cup spinach

½ teaspoon cilantro

½ cup cranberries

1 cup of water

Ice cubes

Directions

- Add all the ingredients to the blender.

- Blend until smooth.
- Serve chilled.

Spicy Tomato Juice

Ingredients

Four large tomatoes

Two tablespoons lemon zest

½ teaspoon basil

½ teaspoon parsley

One teaspoon honey

½ cup of water

Ice cubes

Directions

- Place all the ingredients and blend at high speed.
- Serve chilled.

Banana Milk

Ingredients

Two large bananas

1 cup full cream milk

½ teaspoon cilantro

Ice cubes

Directions

- Place all ingredients in a food processor.
- Blitz at high speed.
- Serve chilled.

Bloody Mary Juice

Ingredients

Three large tomatoes

½ lime, peeled

½ teaspoon hot sauce

½ teaspoon Worcestershire sauce

Dash of salt

Ice cubes

Directions

- Place all the ingredients to a food processor.
- Blitz at high speed.
- Serve chilled.

Green Garden Mix

Ingredients

Four large tomatoes

One small onion, chopped

One tablespoon parsley, fresh

One teaspoon Worcestershire sauce

½ cup kale

½ cup spinach

½ cup sweet bell green pepper

One medium sized carrot, cubed

One tablespoon cilantro, fresh

½ cup of water

Ice cubes

Directions

- Add all ingredients to the blender.
- Blitz at high speed.
- Serve chilled.

Hot Veggie Mix

Ingredients

¼ cup zucchini

½ cup green peas, steamed

¼ cup spinach

¼ cup kale

One small onion, chopped

1 cup full cream yogurt

One tablespoon honey

One teaspoon chipotle

½ cup of water

Ice cubes

Directions

- Place all the ingredients in the blender.
- Blitz at high speed.
- Serve chilled.

Heart Warming Veggie Mix

Ingredients

1 cup beef broth

½ sweet red bell pepper

½ cup carrots, cubed

1 cup kale

Two large tomatoes

One teaspoon Worcestershire sauce

One tablespoon lemon zest

½ teaspoon paprika

½ cup green peas, steamed

One small onion, sliced

1 cup hot water

Directions

- Place your ingredients into the food processor.
- Blend for 2 -3 minutes.
- Serve immediately.

Mango Joy

Ingredients

1 cup mango, unpeeled slices

One large banana, ripe

One tablespoon lemon zest, fresh

½ cup mixed berries

½ cup prunes

½ cup orange juice, fresh

Ice cubes

Directions

- Place all the ingredients into the food blender
- Blend for 1 – 2 minutes.
- Serve chilled.

Pineapple Drink

3 cups pineapple chunks

One tablespoon honey

Ice cubes

Directions

- Place the pineapple, honey and ice cubes into the blender.
- Blend at high speed to 2 – 3 minutes.
- Serve chilled.

Vanilla Banana Shake

One large banana

1 cup mixed berries, frozen

One teaspoon vanilla extract

1 cup full cream milk

One tablespoon cocoa powder

One tablespoon honey

One teaspoon lemon zest

Ice cubes

Directions

- Add the ingredients to the food processor.
- Blend at high speed for 2 minutes.
- Serve chilled.

Kale Cocktail

Ingredients

1 cup kale

½ cup cucumber

½ cup pineapple

Three fresh mint leaves

½ cup of water

Ice cubes

Directions

- Introduce all the elements to the blender.
- Blend for 1 -2 minutes.
- Serve chill.

CHAPTER SEVEN
ECLECTIC SLOW COOKER

Pumpkin Veggie Chipotle

Ingredients

4 cups pumpkin, cubed

Two red bell pepper, sliced

6 cups vegetable broth

One large onion, thinly sliced

Two cloves garlic, minced

1 cup yellow corn

One tablespoon chipotle

Five large tomatoes, quartered

One teaspoon cayenne

3 cups brown beans

2 ½ teaspoon paprika

One teaspoon oregano

One tablespoon cilantro

Sea salt

Directions

- Add all the ingredients to a slow cooker.
- Cook on low heat settings for 7 – 9 hours.
- Serve warm with choice of toppings.

Butter Squash Chili

3 cups lentils

2 cups pureed butter squash

Four cloves garlic, minced

One teaspoon cumin

One green bell pepper, sliced

One large onion, thinly sliced

1 ½ cup vegetable broth

One tablespoon parsley, fresh

One teaspoon oregano

Two tablespoons extra virgin olive oil

One teaspoon jalapeno

Sea salt

Directions

- Add some olive oil to a large saucepan.
- Sauté the onions and garlic for 1 minute.
- Add the lentils, stir and cook for 3 minutes.
- Add the broth and butter squash and stir.
- Add the spices and other ingredients.
- Introduce the contents of the pan into a slow cooker.
- Cook on low heat setting for 5 – 7 hours.
- Serve warm and enjoy!

Cauliflower and Creamy Potato Soup

Ingredients

3 cups beef broth

8 cups full cream milk

1 cup green peas

One small carrot, chopped

Six large potatoes, cubed

Three cloves garlic, minced

One green bell pepper, sliced

Three tablespoons unsalted butter

1 pound cauliflower

3 cups heavy cream

12 ounces cheddar cheese

One teaspoon cayenne

½ teaspoon oregano

½ teaspoon cumin

Sea salt

Directions

- Add the potatoes, butter, and broth to the slow cooker.

- Next, introduce the cauliflower, green peas and carrots.
- Stir the ingredients well.
- Add the cream, spices, milk and stir again.
- Seal the pot and cook on low heat setting for 7 – 9 hours.
- Pour some of the contents of the slow cooker into a high powered food processor.
- Blend until smooth.
- Pour the contents of the blender back to the slow cooker.
- Stir well.
- Cook for 20 minutes on medium heat.
- Serve warm.

Brussels sprout, Pork Chops, and Tomato Soup

Ingredients

Eight bone-in pork chops

2 cups Brussels sprouts

6 cups chicken broth

1 cup kale, chopped

Six large tomatoes, quartered

One large onion, thinly sliced

One tablespoon extra virgin olive oil

One teaspoon chili

One teaspoon basil

One teaspoon parsley

One teaspoon oregano

1 cup carrots, cubed

Sea salt

Directions

- Add the ingredients to the slow cooker.
- Seal the pot.
- Cook on low heat setting for 7 – 9 hours.

- Add the parsley, kale, and basil. Cook for another 10 minutes.
- Serve warm and enjoy!

Hanoi Sirloin and Red Cabbage

Ingredients

2 pounds lean beef sirloin, cubed

Three tablespoons soy sauce

One head red cabbage washed and chopped

Five cloves garlic, minced

One tablespoon ginger, grated

Four tablespoons oyster sauce

One teaspoon baking soda

Two tablespoons cornstarch

Three tablespoons extra virgin olive oil

One large onion, sliced

Three tablespoons brown sugar

One teaspoon cilantro

One tablespoon apple cider vinegar

½ teaspoon paprika

One teaspoon black pepper

Sea salt

Directions

- Combine the vinegar, olive oil, oyster sauce, black pepper, soy sauce, garlic, brown sugar, and ginger.
- To another bowl, add the baking soda, cornstarch, sugar, salt, and water. Combine very well.
- Coat the beef with cornstarch mixture.
- Grease the slow cooker with cooking spray.
- Place the beef in the cooker.
- Pour in the sauce.
- Cook on low heat setting for 5 – 6 hours.
- Add in the red cabbage and stir.

- Cook for 2 minutes.
- Serve warm with pasta or rice.

Pheasant, Carrot and Quinoa Stew

Ingredients

1 pound skinless pheasant legs

6 cups chicken broth

1 cup scallions

2 cups carrots, cubed

1 cup quinoa

½ teaspoon cayenne

1 cup celery, cubed

Two cloves garlic, minced

½ teaspoon curry

½ teaspoon thyme

1 cup black-eyed peas

Sea salt

Directions

- Arrange the pheasant legs on the bottom of the slow cooker.
- Arrange other ingredients in the pot.
- Pour in the broth.
- Seal the pot and cook on low heat setting for 6 – 8 hours.
- Remove the pheasant legs and shred with a fork.
- Add the bird meat back to the pot and stir well.
- Cook on high heat setting for 5 minutes.
- Serve immediately.

Havana Oceana View Stew

Ingredients

1 pound tuna

½ pound prawn, cleaned and peeled

Two tablespoons extra virgin olive oil

Three large tomatoes, quartered

1 cup scallions, chopped

3 cups vegetable broth

Four cloves garlic, minced

One teaspoon oregano

½ teaspoon soy sauce

Two large sweet potatoes, peeled and cubed

½ teaspoon nutmeg

One green bell pepper, sliced

One bay leaf

1 cup green peas

½ teaspoon cumin

Sea salt

Directions

- Sauté the scallions and garlic in olive oil over medium heat for 2 minutes.
- Add the bell pepper and cook for a further 3 minutes.
- Introduce the other spices, stir continuously and cook for 1 minute.
- Pour in the content of the saucepan into a slow cooker.
- Add in the potatoes, tomatoes, green peas, bay leaf, and broth.
- Combine well and cook on high heat setting for 3 – 4 hours.
- Add the tuna and prawns and stir well to combine thoroughly.
- Cook on high heat setting for another 25 – 35 minutes.
- Serve warm and enjoy!

Turkey Wings Burrito Serving

Ingredients

2 pounds boneless, skinless turkey breasts

1 cup diced green chilies

1 cups brown beans

1 cup yellow corn

Two tablespoons taco seasoning

Four large tomatoes, quartered

1 cup cilantro, chopped

One large onion, thinly sliced

Two cloves garlic, minced

1 cup of salsa

Two tablespoons extra virgin olive oil

½ teaspoon nutmeg

Sea salt

Wild rice, cooked

Directions

- First, lay the turkey breasts on the bottom of the slow cooker.

- Add the spices, onions, garlic, corn and brown beans.
- Add the salsa and other ingredients.
- Seal the pot and cook on low heat setting for 7 – 9 hours.
- Pour in the cilantro and stir.
- Serve warm with already prepared wild rice.

Other Books by the Author

The Heavenly Bowls of Buddha Goodness: Mindful Cooking Recipes for Weight Loss, Healthy Living, and Mindful Eating

These Buddha Bowl recipes are not just the trending food in town; it is what your body needs and your tongue craves for at all times. A Buddha Bowl is the agglomeration of a single bowl of delicious and healthy food ingredients. It is a dish based on a balanced combination of vegetables, grains, and proteins. These food classes are not just to be obtained from any source; they should be from organic and life-giving sources that are in peace with the environment and your body.

The term Buddha Bowl tends to elicit a picture of a vegan which is most often the case. However, the recipes cater to the needs of non-vegan individuals too. In as a lot of us are becoming more conscious of our health and eating habits, some persons who seek enlightenment through the way of Buddha will find this book exceptional helpful in meeting their nutritional requirements.

The combination of ingredients ranging from fish, meat to vegetables and grains for the Bowls is almost infinite. This is as a result of the diverse cultures and individual preferences when it comes to how the Bowl is put together. It doesn't matter what your food orientation is, there is something for you. A Buddha Bowl is very easy to prepare with quite a lot of the components requiring little or no cooking.

This book will guide you in making meals that are mouthwatering and at the same time healthy serving as a bonus for the minimal time you spent in preparing it. There is never a dull moment with putting together a Buddha Bowl and enjoying the meal with loved ones.

Are you ready to cleanse your body with some soul-lifting food?

Are you ready to walk away from junk and polluting foods?

Do you think it is time you begin to care for the health of your body?

Looking out for those around you who you genuinely care for?

Then it is time you get this book and lovingly put the recipes and meals together for a healthy and fun filled life.

The Cannabis Cookbook Bible 3 Books in 1: Marijuana Stoner Chef Cookbook, The Healing Path with Essential CBD oil and Hemp oil 32 Delicious Cannabis infused drinks

Considering cooking with cannabis or making use of products of marijuana must have crossed your mind a few times but getting started has been an uphill task with the legal issues surrounding the use of the product. This is not an option as the ignorance, and strict hold on the availability of this plant has been eased gradually. With the regulations appearing to come to terms with the inevitability of making mainstream cannabis use, you can fully start to enjoy the amazing benefits of cannabis and its allied products.

This book is a compilation of three books; The Healing Path with Essential CBD oil and Hemp oil; The Simple Beginners Guide to Managing Anxiety Attacks, Weight Loss, Diabetes and Holistic Healing, 32 Delicious Cannabis infused drinks; Healthy marijuana appetizers, tonics, and cocktails and Marijuana Stoner Chef Cookbook A Beginners Guide to Simple, Easy and Healthy Cannabis Recipes. These books were written to start you on the path of living a healthy life free of pain and everyday discomforts, having a delicious meal with friends and family and spicing up your day.

What other reasons do you need to buy this book?

- You get a beginners idea of what cannabis is all about
- How to buy high-grade marijuana.
- Know the great health benefits you can get from the use of cannabis and CBD oil.
- Great recipes and edibles that you can make from cannabis.
- Guide on how to dose using CBD oil.
- How to maximize the effects of cannabis in your cooking.
- Preparing cannabis-infused smoothies, cocktails and beverages that can be made from cannabis.

This book is all you need to become comfortable and have a nice relation making use of cannabis. This is a plant that can be incorporated into your everyday meals. You will also learn how you can explore this plant and derive the very best it has got to offer.

You have waited your whole life for this very moment. Don't let his minute slip by you. Get this book now explore the colorful world of cannabis!

The Healing Path with Essential CBD oil and Hemp oil: The Simple Beginner's Guide to Managing Anxiety Attacks, Weight Loss, Diabetes and Holistic Healing

Suffering from arthritis, diabetes, severe chronic pain and a host of other debilitating ailments can limit your quality of life. The constant intake of a cocktail of medications will always leave you with horrible aftermaths that were not listed on the package of such drugs. The battering and deterioration that your internal organs undergo can only just be imagined as these medications cause more damage than good in the long run.

The wholesome nature and abundant benefits that CBD oil has cannot just be overlooked. Its uses range from managing common pains and to the more complex and debilitating conditions that ravage us in this age and time. It is used for the treatment of pains, depression, irritable bowel syndrome, epilepsy and illnesses that you can never imagine will be easily handled by this compound. CBD is wholly naturally without any hint of synthetic compounds is just what you need for that immediate relief from the condition that has been keeping you down for so long.

This book is a beginner guide on what CBD and Hemp oil are, all you need to know, some of the numerous ailments that it can be used to treat, modes of preparation, how to dose on CBD and a guide of how to shop for CBD. Also addressed in this book is the nagging issues of legal barriers that are continually being surmounted with each passing day as new information on the benefits of CBD oil comes to light.

Are you ready to know how you can use CBD oil to;

- Boost your immune system
- Have a clearer skin
- Control those pains
- Increase your sexual appetite
- Lighten your moods
- Have a good night's rest
- Improve your learning and retention abilities
- And have a generally healthy and wholesome lifestyle?

In this beginner's guide, you will be made aware of how CBD oil can be the best thing that ever happened to you.

So for how long are you going to cope with that pain, the condition that keeps you down most of the day? Take that all critical, decisive step now, dump the medications that are not doing you any good and embrace the natural path to healing.

Get this book now!

Cannabis Bud Smoothie: Healthy Medicinal Drinks and Marijuana Infusions

Quite a lot of folks with chronic medical conditions are sceptical about the consumption of marijuana by smoking it. If you are in this category, then here is an easy way out. Taking in medicinal cannabis by adding it to your delicious smoothies and juicing it will give you all the health benefits and much more! Ingesting of cannabis fresh and raw is the most advantageous as all the nutrients, and cannabinoid compounds will remain intact without undergoing any change into compounds that you may not necessarily need at this point.

You will learn how to incorporate cannabis buds and cannabis infusions into your daily smoothies to aid you in managing those severe pains, inflammations, ailments and generally giving you a more healthy life.

This book is filled with a delicious smoothie, and juice recipes packed loaded with vitamins, nutrients and cannabinoids. The recipes are organic, gluten and sugar-free with the foundation been cannabis.

In this book, you will learn;

- The great health benefits of cannabis How to prepare delicious smoothies and juices
- Ease away those excruciating pains And so much more!

BUY this book today and begin your journey towards a more healthier life!

Cannabis Cultivation and Horticulture: The Simple Guide to Growing Marijuana Indoors Using Hydroponics

This is an excellent guide for beginners and professionals alike on the indoor cultivation of marijuana for personal use using hydroponics and soil. It brings to you the simple techniques and methods need to have a thriving sanctuary for your cannabis plants and produce plants with potent buds and massive amounts of resins! Cultivating your cannabis indoors gives you the opportunity to monitor its growth and make adjustments to the environmental conditions that will significantly stimulate the growth of the plant. It is also an avenue to prevent the pestilence that comes with outdoor cultivation. Looking to have a basic knowledge that can be leveraged to grow great plants? Then this is the book for you!

Major and minor parts involved in the cultivation of cannabis are thoroughly handled. From the design and type of sanctuary space to the kind of nutrients, lightning to temperature, pest control to flow of air; everything you need to grow potent strains of marijuana is just within your grasp. Each stage of cultivation from obtaining the seeds to drying and curing is fully explained in terms that you can easily understand and put to practice immediately. So do you want to take the first steps towards nurturing this beautiful plant from seed to a potent wonder of nature? This book will teach you how to

- Grow your stash while employing high safety standards
- Learn how to secure a discrete growing space in a confined area
- Have the ability to determine the potency of your product
- Force flowering
- Applying the best nutrients formulas to

your plants
- Crossing and identifying the best strain for you
- Getting all unfertilized female plants (Sensimilla)
- Controlling Pests
- Making the best use of the hydroponics
- And so much more!

Getting started with this book will make you an enlightened cultivator and appreciator of everything cannabis and not just a grower. BUY this book now and have a high time!

The Complete Instant Pot Cookbook: Simple Ketogenic Diet Cookbook Recipes, The Simple Slow Cooker Cookbook and The Healthy Crock Pot Cookbook

This amazing collection of books will take you on a journey of culinary delights that you can put together with ease. Coming home to a well cooked, a stomach-warming meal will now be the norm for you and your household. With quite a number of great recipes to choose from you will be absolutely spoilt with choices.

Lay your hand on this volume of healthy crockpot and instant pot recipes for the price of one. You will never have a shortage of recipes you can try out at any given time ranging from desserts to main dishes and chili to exotic recipes.

You will not just be getting mouth-watering recipes, also included are guidelines on what to look out for when you want to buy a crockpot, healthy tips on going on a ketogenic diet plan and so much more!

What are you waiting for? Do not let this opportunity slip by you. GET this book NOW and also as a gift for your loved ones.

About the Author

Rina S. Gritton has been all about healthy intake of food and living the life of a real food aficionado. With her it is about food, making us of spices, herbs, and other ingredients around in nature that ensures we all stay at the peak of our health at all times.

She has been putting together great recipes and meals as a hobby and business to loved ones and clients alike. What started as a challenge to help her parents and siblings eat better turned to a full-fledged campaign and career in making use of purely organic foods and materials around us.

A dietician with several years experience in the treatment of dietary issues and business owner catering for the desires of folks to have organic and tasteful meals, she also guest writes for blogs, websites, and volunteers in cooking classes in high schools.

She lives in Santa Monica, California with her husband and children.